2/2'

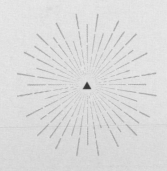

THE
POWER
AGE

THE
POWER
AGE

Kelly Doust

Illustrated by JESSICA GUTHRIE

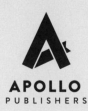

APOLLO
PUBLISHERS

DEDICATED TO BELINDA,
WHOSE OWN POWER AGE ENDED TOO SOON.

CONTENTS

INTRODUCTION

YOUR
SECOND ACT

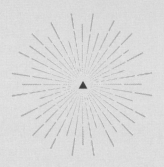

From a very early age I always wanted to be old. Or older, at least. Age seemed to me to confer the attributes that made life worth living, and which childhood and adolescence sorely missed. Being older meant two things to me: experience and freedom, and I wanted them both so badly I could almost scream.

Now, when I discuss this with my eleven-year-old daughter, she hoots with laughter at the thought of growing up, screwing up her freckled nose in distaste. She loves being a kid. When I ask her why, she says that being an adult is 'boring and stressful', and she's right in one respect: it does come hand-in-hand with some fairly annoying downsides, like mortgages and divorce, and routine colonoscopies, and realising that your face takes at least several hours to wake up after you do (gone, your dewy-faced visage, replaced with skin that seems to crease like origami paper when you sleep). But that makes the moments of joy more prized and sweet. Life has greater poignancy when you realise there's less of it to live with each passing year.

Our culture positively deifies youth — you need only look at Instagram to see that, or clock that most of the models in fashion magazines are still in their teens. Someone set the match with rock 'n' roll and the Youth Quake of the 1960s, and the young things have been burning brightly ever since.

Thank goodness, the tide finally seems to be turning. Because being in the later years of your life has never looked so good. The World Health Organization agrees, calling population ageing 'one of humanity's greatest triumphs'. But it is the *way* in which modern women are redefining themselves as they grow older that is most thrilling for those approaching — or well into the swing of — midlife themselves.

Being older is different to the way it was fifty, or even twenty, years ago. Your Nan's voluminous flowered housedress? A thing of the past. Sitting on the porch whistling and watching the world go by? I don't think so. Women middle-aged and older are *killing* it. Some look like Ari Seth Cohen's cool and kooky *Advanced Style* cohorts. Others cock two fingers at the establishment before they'll conform to anyone's idea of femininity, and are all the better for it. (Dame Vivienne Westwood, Oprah and Patti Smith, we're looking at you.)

Women over fifty are amongst the most successful of today's entrepreneurs, but they're also the fastest-growing group of homeless people in otherwise affluent nations, so it's not all bread and roses. With the anti-anti-ageing trend in full swing, and older women in particular more visible than ever in public life, things are changing — and they sorely needed to. We are in more positions of power than ever before. It's about time. The legacy this is leaving for younger women is profound and world-shifting.

I remember the phrase 'Don't wish your life away', trotted out whenever I was itching with impatience to do those things considered well beyond my years. Because youth is everything, especially for a woman, or so we're told. We're in the prime of our

'Being older is different to the way it was fifty, or even twenty, years ago.'

▲

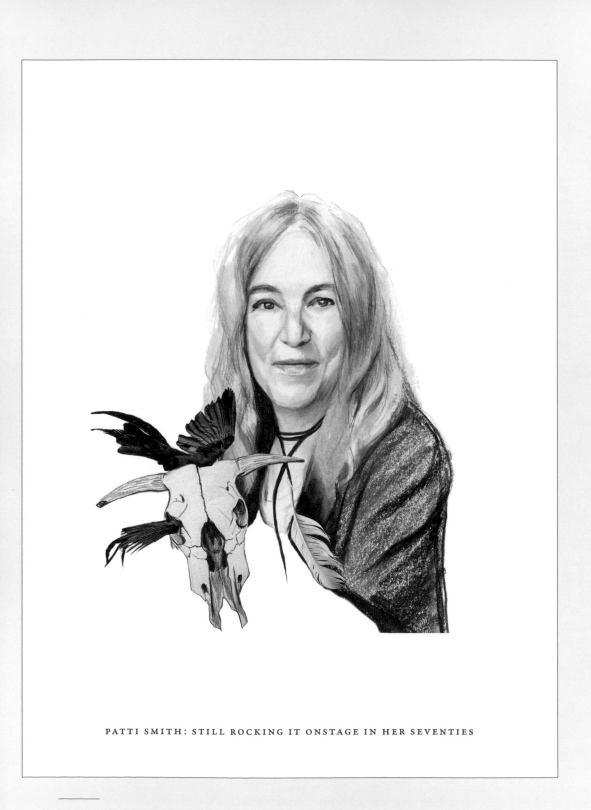

PATTI SMITH: STILL ROCKING IT ONSTAGE IN HER SEVENTIES

lives until we hit 35 (some would say younger, as Picasso did of his 17-year-old lover, Marie-Thérèse Walter, when he was 42!), then it's all downhill from there. We know this for the absolute rubbish it is, and yet the youth bias persists.

Now that I've hit my forties, and am starting to step into my own 'power age', I can tell you that what I long suspected is true: being a grown woman is more than it's cracked up to be (well, most of the time). Entering your second act is not so scary as it once seemed. In fact, it can be pretty fabulous. It's truly exciting to find out who you are and evolve into the person you were always meant to be. This is a journey of unfolding that simply can't happen overnight. It takes years and years of trial and error, and life lessons, and loss, to come home to ourselves and figure out who we are, what inspires us, and what makes us tick. A few wrinkles and saggy bits seem a paltry compromise for this treasure chest full of riches.

There's something quite depressing about those who are desperate to hold onto their youth. Of course there are things to mourn as we get older, but it seems sad to focus on what we've lost, rather than what we have also gained. I have noticed the ageing process in my own body, but am happier than I've ever been, and more comfortable in my own skin. Becoming stuck on the external is to miss the point of why we're here. But retaining a youthful sense of vigour and curiosity about the world around us will never go out of style or look ridiculous. Indeed, they are two of the most vital elements to ageing well.

Not all older people are wise, and there are younger souls who possess wisdom well beyond their years, but I have sought the advice of wise older women for as long as I can remember. 'The One Who Knows, old La Que Sabe, The Wild Woman', as Clarissa Pinkola Estés calls them in *Women Who Run With the Wolves*. Women who have shared with me so many nuggets of truth, and provided a template for the sort of woman I wish to

'Entering your second act is not so scary as it once seemed.'

▲

Your
Second Act

become. I look to them for inspiration, wondering what guides them, about the experiences that have shaped their lives, and the sort of imprint they hope to leave on the world when they're gone. I'm interested to know what they think holds the most meaning, and consider the lives they've built and choices they've made like a student, all the while trying to make sense of my own desire to cultivate a life less ordinary. I love these women fiercely for showing me the way — to a journey of becoming underpinned by true passion and fearlessness.

I was looking for this book long before I decided to write it. Where was the alternative narrative, I wondered? The one that asserted it's great to grow old and step into your power? Not just great, but *the best*. So many of us fall prey to the idea that we need to stay young, but the very best women have always worn their vintage with pride and welcomed new adventures with open arms, even in decline.

And so this book, *The Power Age*, is intended as a celebration of growing older, and being an older woman in particular, and the ways in which we can embrace this inevitable process — loving and nurturing ourselves through our fifties, sixties and beyond, and realising how precious this phase of life is, in its complexity, hardship and joy. I've struck up conversations and sought sage advice from women I admire to share with you here, and included their thoughts and tips on a whole range of subjects to hopefully help you confirm that you're on the right path, or to provide you with the support you need to find your way.

Because you are not alone, and you are not invisible. Your voice is important and it needs to be heard. So shout it from the rooftops, and welcome your own power age.

If not now, then when?

A great life is here for the taking, always. There are so many opportunities, if we only open our eyes and hearts to them.

And it is never, ever too late.

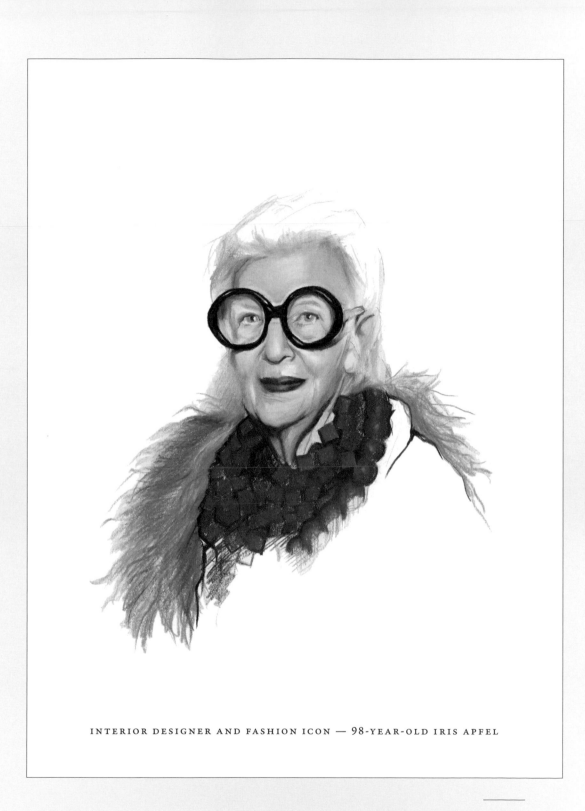

INTERIOR DESIGNER AND FASHION ICON — 98-YEAR-OLD IRIS APFEL

You are never too old for ...

- ▶ Love
- ▶ A new direction
- ▶ A signature scent
- ▶ Becoming more self-aware
- ▶ Finding work that fulfils you
- ▶ Compassion
- ▶ Making a new friend
- ▶ Educating yourself
- ▶ Fabulous costume jewellery and accessories
- ▶ Childlike wonder
- ▶ Developing your witty repartee
- ▶ Emotional intelligence
- ▶ Honing your sense of style
- ▶ Taking care of yourself
- ▶ Writing a memoir
- ▶ Appreciating all the beauty in the world around us

Retirement is not in the vocabulary

Q&A WITH HELEN CLARK,
FORMER PRIME MINISTER OF NEW ZEALAND

▲

Helen Clark, 69, is the second woman to hold the post and fifth-longest serving prime minister. She was also the first female head of the United Nations Development Programme.

How has it been stepping down from Parliament and the United Nations, and what's next for you?

It's felt liberating after half a century in institutions — first the University of Auckland, then Parliament, then the United Nations. Now I choose exactly what I want to do and when I do it. I'm ticking things off the bucket list, like taking the Trans-Siberian Railway and visiting Mozambique, and my husband has been working with a board of trustees to set up a foundation in my name. The idea is to support and work around things I've long been interested in, such as evidence-based policy, public health and penal policy.

I found that even after I left the United Nations, the emails and phone calls never stopped coming. I ended up being very busy with various advisory boards, events, lectures and keynote speeches. Especially because I don't specialise in any one thing — I'm involved in sustainability and the environment, HIV and sexually transmitted diseases, a whole range of women's issues, and

Your
Second Act

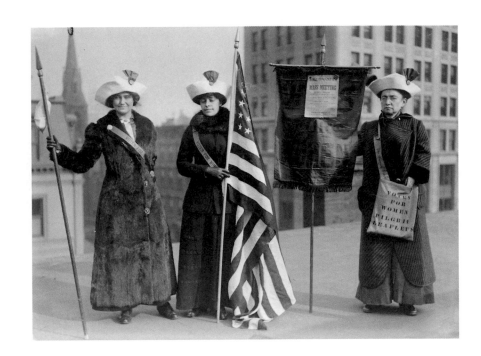

FIGHTING FOR EMANCIPATION, THE EARLY SUFFRAGETTES
HELPED PAVE THE WAY FOR EQUALITY

drug policy, amongst others. This all conspires to keep me quite busy. Retirement is not in the vocabulary. But a lot of people of my generation stay active. Just stopping and hanging up your boots at 65 is almost unthinkable.

New Zealand has a history of better equality for women than many Western nations. Why do you think that is?
We're a small country but when movements get traction here, they tend to sweep nationwide. We were not a rich colony, but a society where European settler women worked just as hard as men did. In the early 1890s when the first suffragettes pushed for the vote, they set the tone for other New Zealand women. It took a while, but it laid the groundwork for others to push on through.

What would be your number one piece of advice for women in mid-to-late life?
I guess it depends on what they've been involved in, and whether they are able to carry on. I'm very conscious that there's a difference in my life to a woman who's been standing on a factory floor for four decades — I can understand if she would like to take a rest and wind down. We all come from different contexts.

For women who have been professional like myself, there is no reason to stop. There is a lot to be done out there on a pro-bono basis. Think of all the women coming out of medicine, law, business and other industries that are crying out for board members. There's teaching, or considering the other inspiring things women do in their later years. There are always community-based initiatives looking for people to help.

Get involved where you feel you can make a difference.

What does power mean to you?
Power in itself is a neutral concept — I think it can be put to good or bad ends, and I like to think I put it into doing good.

For me, it's about having the platform to build a better, happier, healthier and more inclusive society which is considerate of nature and the environment.

How do you hope people will remember you, and what do you think will be your legacy?
I put a lot of effort into making things different for people and supporting them — I'd like to think I was ahead of my time in this respect. In my years of being Prime Minister there were a lot of good policies put into place, and a lot of things have endured. I had a vision for a better New Zealand. I'd like to think I was someone who put the building blocks in place for defining our values, developing our culture and the arts, and supporting families, which reaped dividends for generations.

You certainly paved the way for Jacinda Ardern (New Zealand's current female Prime Minister — the youngest woman ever in the role and the first to give birth while in the post).
We all stand on the shoulders of those who came before, and those 1893 suffragettes were the first example.

Lastly, what would you say to older women who feel they are invisible or don't have a voice in current society?
It's shocking that people are living in a context where that's how they perceive they are seen. Self-esteem is incredibly important, and anything one can do to encourage self-worth. Your voice and engagement *is* important. Don't just pack it all away and think that's the end. We can expect to have long lives. Find things that stir your passion — this could be family or local organisations. Don't wait to be asked, just crash on in. I don't think anyone ever rolled out a red carpet for me. Find resilience and self-esteem, and roll out the red carpet for yourself!

'Find resilience and self-esteem, and roll out the red carpet for yourself!'

▲

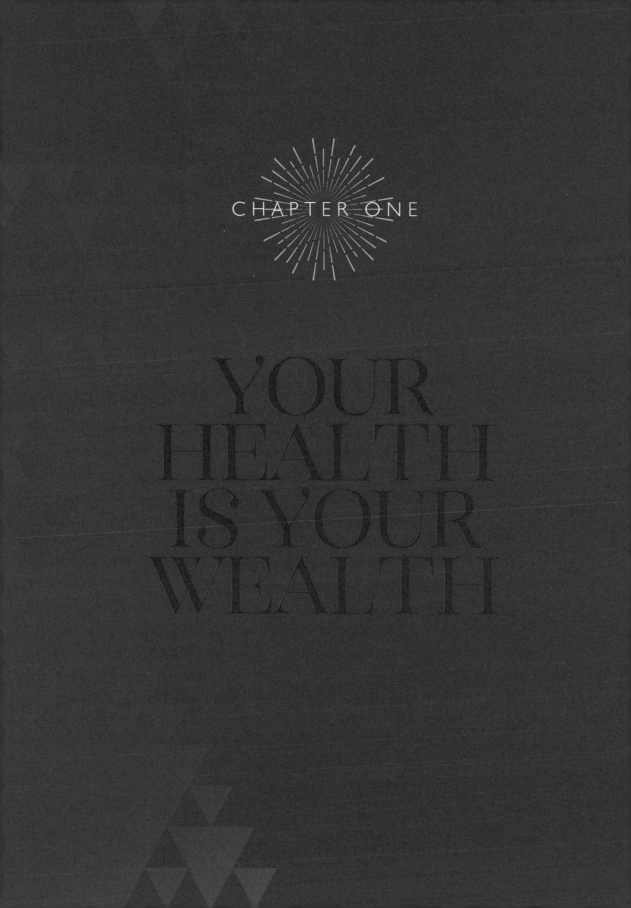

CHAPTER ONE

YOUR HEALTH IS YOUR WEALTH

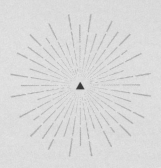

Enjoying great health is everything. It gives us the energy to get through the day and pursue the things we dream of doing, and it's the number one foundation for a good life. Many of us are so conscious of our health nowadays. We're living longer, generally staying fit and active much later in life than our parents and grandparents did, and have access to a fabulously wide, varied diet. If we don't fall prey to excess or stress — the top two life-shorteners beyond major illness or misadventure — we are, generally, laughing through the home strait.

But not so much as some centenarians. From a study of 'Blue Zone' areas (those parts of the world where people don't just live longer, but seem to thrive and enjoy a better quality of life well into their dotage), it's clear that the tenets for a good life are simple: spend heaps of time outdoors in fresh air doing incidental exercise, cultivate close friendships, get enough sleep, and generally live a pared-back existence with few possessions or worries. Blue Zone residents also eat a lighter, more nutritious diet than many of us — but it's not so much *what* they eat as the *way* they eat it, creating a ritual of appreciation around food by taking time out to enjoy their meals.

Modern life is fast-moving, and we can't all move to Sardinia or Japan, so how to incorporate more island-style living into the everyday?

Creating a strong foundation

While it's impossible to prevent health issues from cropping up now and then, we can give our body the best possible chance, both for ageing well and for recovering when issues do arise. Here's a list of basic, sensible wellness tips to remember when you're feeling out of whack.

▸ **Stress less.** It's easier said than done, but consider the main stressors in your life and work to remove them, or at least change your reaction when they do occur. You're only as stressed as you allow yourself to be. Overwhelm and anxiety often come from taking on too much, so try to shift some things off your plate and notice the difference.

▸ **Eat fresh, nutritious whole foods.** Try to find high-quality, ethically produced meat or other protein, and steer clear of too much salt and sugar. Eat organic and non-genetically modified foods when you can, and don't overeat. Aim for feeling satisfied after a meal rather than uncomfortably full, and your gut will love you for it. Better digestion = happier humans.

▸ **Keep up your daily exercise.** Even if it's just a walk around the block, a quick swim or dancing around the house to your favourite tunes when you get dressed in the morning. Our bodies are built to move. They don't work so well when we stop.

▸ **Do weight training.** This builds bone density and can make a difference to your health at any age. Body-weight exercises work, but lifting weights is even better. You don't need to make like a CrossFit champion — smaller weights focusing on steady, controlled repetitions work just as well for building bone density and muscle, and helping you stay strong into your later years.

Your Health Is
Your Wealth

▸ **Stay hydrated.** It's said we humans are made up of around 90 percent water, so basically we're just watermelons with brains. Poor hydration leads to lower brain function, tiredness, and in severe cases to a raft of other health issues, such as kidney stones.

▸ **Sleep, perchance to dream.** Did you know insomnia, sleep apnea and other sleep issues have a huge impact, not just on your health but your general wellbeing? A solid eight hours per night (or seven, in a pinch) helps your body and cells repair themselves. Guard your horizontal hours like the precious resource they are.

▸ **Watch for signs of chronic anxiety and mental health issues.** Women suffer from higher anxiety rates than men, and this increases in middle life when work and family responsibilities tend to pile up. Make sure you have a 'pressure valve' to let off steam when you need to, and do more of whatever makes you feel happy. Maybe it's a night out singing karaoke with friends, or a weekend away at a health spa. Maybe it's simply carving out enough downtime for yourself to unplug from devices and truly unwind. Curl up on the sofa with a good novel. Take the dog for a walk. Do your nails. Just make sure you take regular time out when you feel the pressure building, or even visit your GP to discuss. If it all gets too much, don't be afraid to seek professional help: there is so much support available these days, and far less stigma around these issues than there used to be.

How would you like to look and feel?

When figuring out which sport or activity you'd like to pursue, look at the shape of those who do it regularly. Fancy a dancer's physique? Try barre classes in your spare time. Like the long, toned thighs of a Pilates instructor? Sign up for a session. Always admired Madonna's toned upper arms? Take up weight lifting. Treat your body like a temple, but don't take it all too seriously. Everything in moderation, including moderation.

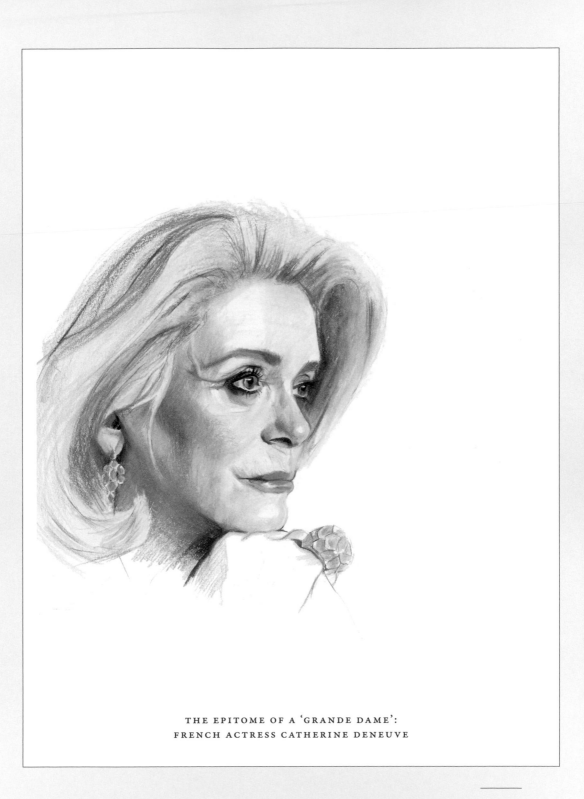

THE EPITOME OF A 'GRANDE DAME':
FRENCH ACTRESS CATHERINE DENEUVE

Get bendy

Yoga crops up quite a lot throughout this book. That's because so many women in their power age seem to be at it, or recommend yoga as one of their top activities for staying calm and fit.

No matter what your health situation or past injuries are, chances are you can still do a modified form of yoga — even if it's simply yin, a gentle stretching class said to replenish a person's physical and mental reserves.

There are over 100 different types of yoga being practised today, but most sessions typically include gentle breathing exercises, a series of holding postures (sometimes called *asana*, or poses) for varying lengths of time, as well as a few minutes of meditation towards the end of the class.

The American Osteopathic Association says maintaining a regular yoga practice can provide a range of physical benefits:

- ▶ increased flexibility
- ▶ increased muscle strength and tone
- ▶ improved breathing, energy and vitality
- ▶ maintaining a balanced metabolism
- ▶ weight reduction
- ▶ maintaining or improving cardio and circulatory health
- ▶ improved athletic performance
- ▶ protection from injury

Through stretching exercises that flex the various muscle groups, yoga is also said to help aid the body in its ability to heal itself, and increase harmony in body and mind, while lessening chronic pain, lowering blood pressure and reducing insomnia.

If you're not already into yoga, give it a go. It can also be a gentle gateway into other healing and stress-relieving modalities, such as meditation.

Positive ageing

INTERVIEW WITH DR. JOANNA MCMILLAN,
NUTRITION AND LIFESTYLE SPECIALIST

▲

Scottish-born Dr. Joanna McMillan, 47, is one of Australia's
best-known nutrition and lifestyle specialists. A PhD-qualified
nutrition scientist, Accredited Practising Dietitian and Adjunct
Senior Research Fellow with La Trobe University, she is also a
Fellow of the Australasian Society of Lifestyle Medicine and a regular
on television and radio, as well as the author of seven books.
In her early career she worked as a qualified fitness instructor,
teaching aerobics and weights classes before deciding to pursue
nutrition. After more than a decade in the public eye,
Joanna understands the pressure to look young and glamorous
as an older woman. Here's her advice for ageing well.

Working in the media, I certainly see women who are so Botox-ed
they can barely move their faces. I totally understand the struggle
so I'm not judging — we are a different generation from our
mothers and grandmothers; we want to age well, age gracefully,
and we want to look and feel our best.

But it's great to be happy and proud of the age you are.
We're a generation of women who don't want to be thought of
as 'middle-aged', and we have the potential to combat premature
ageing through the lifestyle choices we make. These choices —

Your Health Is
Your Wealth

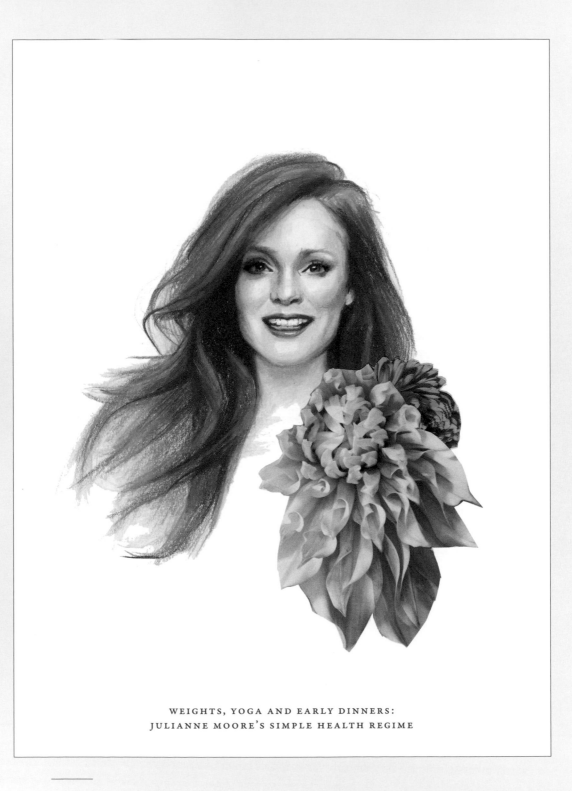

WEIGHTS, YOGA AND EARLY DINNERS:
JULIANNE MOORE'S SIMPLE HEALTH REGIME

particularly pertaining to sleep and stress — make a huge difference. The power of lifestyle medicine is positive ageing.

There are niggles about getting older, but with age also comes a kind of wisdom — experience and credibility and career opportunities. Once we no longer have young children, we should be able to get more sleep, which is essential. And we're usually more advanced in our careers, with the freedom to tailor a career that suits us more.

For me, I really love this age. My kids are older, my career is at a good point, I feel good. We should be caring less about the silly stuff and recognise that getting older also has its benefits.

In terms of the things you can do to add 'years to life and life to years', a plant-rich diet filled with a wealth of different, vital chemicals that will help your skin and body age well is your foundation. It's truly amazing how food can repair cells, DNA and build your brain. If you eat well, it will help your body age as well as possible.

I have a theory that there are six pillars to good health: Food, Drink, Exercise, Activity, Sleep and Stress. Most importantly, all of this should be underpinned by joy. A healthy lifestyle is not a *fait accompli*. It takes balance and mindfulness, and it's never 'done'.

Society reveres the skinny body, but every woman over the age of 35 needs to be doing strength training for their health. I see a lot of women who run to stay thin, but don't focus on weights or building their strength. That's what gets you out of your chair in your older years.

As we age, our body-fat distribution changes, and if you have no muscle, you're much more likely to be frail as an older person and have falls and break bones. Strength is also going to help you in menopause, because with more muscle on your bones you're unlikely to put on as much weight. Start small with strength training, focus on form, and do short reps, and the risk of injury is much lower.

One of the things I've noticed is that we don't talk about the long term enough — fads and certain dietary tribes seem to be

'A healthy lifestyle is not a fait accompli. *It takes balance and mindfulness, and it's never "done".'*

▲

Your Health Is
Your Wealth

———

all about cutting things out of your diet, but it's the foundations you lay and what you do regularly over time that makes the most impact.

It comes down to discipline, and being aware of your own likes and dislikes. It's the same with exercise. Commitment to a 6 am fitness class, for example, reaps rewards over time. Our emphasis should be on health and wellness rather than weight — with no end date in mind.

Dr. Joanna's key foundations for a healthy diet as we age

- Keep it rich in plant foods.
- Eat protein in every meal, spaced out across the day. Prior to menopause women have really high iron requirements, and red meat is a hard-to-beat source. As we get older, our bodies are less efficient at processing protein, and consuming a regular dose helps us utilise it efficiently. Nevertheless, many of us are having way too much protein, and particularly when this occurs without enough fiber, it causes toxic products to form in the gut's microbiome. Beware of consuming protein powders and too many protein supplements, which are processed.
- Check up on calcium. Women in particular need to be careful about their calcium intake and make sure they're getting enough. Without it, our bones become brittle as we age.If you don't consume dairy, you need to introduce calcium-fortified milks into your diet, such as soy or nut milk.
- Get your daily dose of sunshine. With the dangers of skin cancer, many of us are avoiding time in the sun, but this can lead to a deficiency of vitamin D, which is also essential for

bone health. Your body can't make use of calcium without vitamin D, so take supplements if you're really not spending any time outdoors or in sunlight.

- **Adjust your food intake.** It's generally agreed that we need less food as we age, and if your energy levels or needs have changed, take note and recognise that you probably don't need as much food as you once did. This makes it even more important to ensure that the foods you are eating are highly nutritious.

- **Get enough iron.** After menopause, our iron requirements are much lower because we're not losing it through menstruation every month. However, iron is still important post-menopause and beyond, so don't disregard it completely.

- **Enjoy good fats.** We've demonised fats for way too long! Good fats can be found in foods such as avocados and extra virgin olive oil, which contain powerful antioxidants to help with ageing.

- **Eat your carbs, but the good ones found in whole foods.** Bear in mind that most of our fiber comes from carb-containing foods, and with whole grains comes a lower risk of bowel cancer. We take important nutrients from grains, but avoid the refined stuff. Stick to whole foods such as rolled oats, brown rice, quinoa, legumes and whole grain sourdough, and don't put all carbs in the same basket — some are very good for you and give you the energy you need to get through the day. Plus they're good for your brain: a low intake of whole grains has been associated with more inflammation and accelerated cognitive decline with age.

- **Trust your body and listen to your appetite.** Don't be lured by new fads. Consider your allergies and intolerances, your cultural background, and your likes and dislikes.

- **Cultivate a more relaxed relationship with food, and don't forget to introduce that important element: joy!**

Your Health Is
Your Wealth

Managing menopause

INTERVIEW WITH DR. GINNI MANSBERG,
WOMEN'S HEALTH GP AND AUTHOR

▲

Dr. Ginni Mansberg, 50, is a practising GP who specialises
in women's health. A host on TV's *Medicine or Myth* and
Embarrassing Bodies, Ginni is also a regular guest on morning
television and the author of four books on women's health,
including the *The M Word*, all about menopause and
perimenopause. Here's the scoop on navigating
the hormonal rollercoaster.

Traditionally, post-menopause is seen as a good time for women,
where they report being statistically happier. But many women
have a difficult time in their forties and early fifties — the period
known as perimenopause, before menopause even starts.

'Their ovaries are running at a subpar level, hormones go up and
down, and it can really vary from one month to the next, or even one
hour to the next, how women feel during this time,' explains Ginni.

'An excess of estrogen — what I often refer to as the "go-go
hormone" without the balancing effects of progesterone —
means women can have anxiety and trouble sleeping, which can
then lead to anxiety. They often experience heavier periods, too.
Then, when there's a drop in estrogen, symptoms like hot flashes,
vaginal dryness, brain fog and loss of libido can occur, which have

implications for women's relationships or even their career. And it adds a whole new layer of complexity to sleep issues.'

Ginni says eating well, getting enough sleep and exercising all help, but sometimes antidepressants are prescribed to deal with the emotional effects of hormones being all over the place. Perimenopause, she adds, can go on for a decade or more!

Hormone replacement therapy (HRT) or menopausal hormone therapy (MHT, as it's now called) is really the gold standard of treatment for women experiencing hot flashes, aches and pains, vaginal dryness and an increased risk of urinary tract infections. There are alternative therapies, Ginni explains, but none of them is as effective for menopausal symptoms as HRT or MHT medication. 'There are some women who can't take it — if you've had breast cancer, clotting problems, uncontrollable high blood pressure or liver disease, there are contraindications to using the medication. But when you can use it, it can be life changing. It helps women immensely.'

Ginni was appearing on morning television in 2002 the day news broke about the links between breast cancer and HRT, after which scores of women threw their HRT medication in the bin and started seeking alternative remedies. Ginni, however, says the risk of cancer from using HRT is still greatly overstated.

'There is a slightly increased risk of breast cancer for certain women, but no more than when drinking a glass of wine per night. When women drink two glasses of wine per night, the risk is even greater than taking HRT. And research shows that one of the groups taking up drinking this amount the most is menopausal women.'

Your GP won't prescribe MHT if you're not experiencing hot flashes or your symptoms aren't bothering you too much, explains Ginni.

'Once, they used to suggest everyone go on these medications, but it's no longer the case. Natural therapies can have a placebo effect — and as long as the therapy is benign, that can be a good solution.

'Many peak, exacting medical bodies around the world have conducted studies into HRT and MHT, and have concluded that the risks for most women are negligible.'

▲

Your Health Is Your Wealth

But we know many of these products being prescribed are actually *harmful*. There's a lot of pseudoscience around bioidentical hormones, for example, but no evidence to back up that they actually work. Unfortunately, though, they've been marketed very effectively to women who are fearful of using MHT.'

Many peak, exacting medical bodies around the world have conducted studies into HRT and MHT, and have concluded that the risks for most women are negligible, Ginni explains. But some drug companies have stopped producing these medications because the demand for them has decreased. This has made the medications more expensive, says Ginni, especially as there are no longer any government subsidies to keep costs low. Afraid of being sued, GPs are also hesitant to prescribe these medications — all of which means women are not getting the support they need.

'People talk about ageing gracefully or naturally, but post-menopausal women many years ago often died or became dried-up crones,' Ginni points out. 'Can you imagine a man putting up with the same symptoms? Women are conditioned to be carers and put themselves second — but telling them they should simply "put up with it" is misogyny,' she says.

'As women can now expect to live almost half their lives on the other side of menopause, they want to do it in great health and style. We need knowledge to empower us through the journey of hormone hell (perimenopause) and beyond (menopause proper). Plus we want good humor; realistic, achievable remedies; and a sense of collaboration and fun.'

If you're unsure about which treatment to seek, talk with your doctor or contact women's health groups that can provide brilliant information, research and valuable resources for perimenopausal and menopausal women.

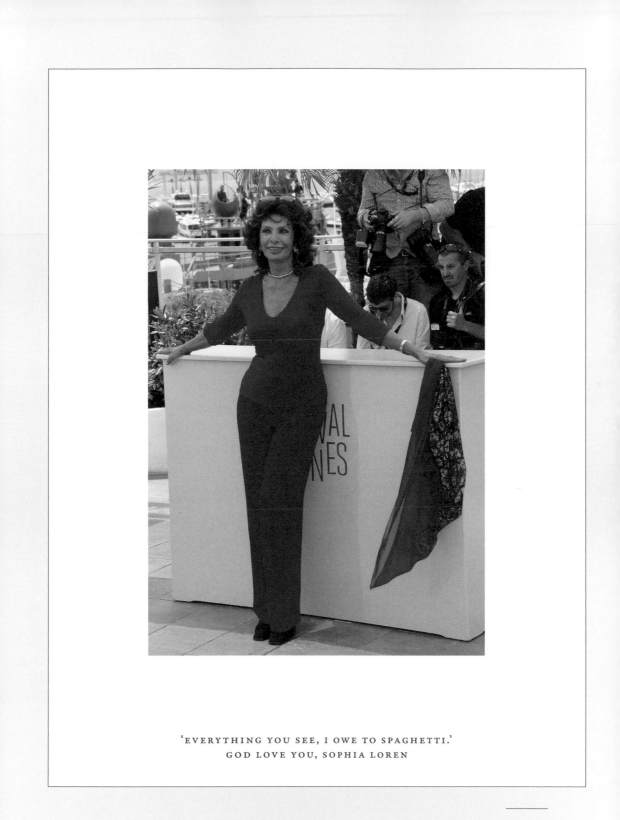

'EVERYTHING YOU SEE, I OWE TO SPAGHETTI.'
GOD LOVE YOU, SOPHIA LOREN

Giving chronic pain a good dose of attitude

Q&A WITH CHELSEA BONNER, FOUNDER OF BELLA MODELS, ONE OF THE WORLD'S LEADING CURVE MODELLING AGENCIES

▲

Chelsea Bonner's book, *Body Image Warrior: One woman's fight for change in the modelling industry*, details her battle with body image issues and chronic poor health as a sufferer of fibromyalgia. Chelsea, 45, recently underwent a hysterectomy and is in recovery.

Women are shown images of unrealistic bodies every day, and you have intimate knowledge of how that's constructed. What have you learned about the relationship between body image and health?
I've learned over many years of working in this field that beauty and self-esteem are completely different things. One's own self-perception is at the core of everything we do, think, wear, learn, and strive for — and our attitude towards body image is no different. We are conditioned from an early age that we will only be *truly* successful if we are also slim and beautiful, and that all other achievements are irrelevant unless you also tick that box. As women it's almost like you are not successful unless you are also considered a beauty. The media and the world around us reinforces that every minute of every day.

I know so many incredible women kicking so many goals that no one ever hears about because they are not considered photogenic enough, which is ridiculous. Think about all the businesswomen you know and who the spotlight is focused on. This message doubles down on the already-imprinted idea that you are not sexy, or fun, or lovable, or even allowed to go on trips to exotic locations unless you are slim. Every single advertisement for every single product you can think of is sold to us through the images of success as being this generation's idea of attractive, prescribed by very clever creatives and brain-mapping studies that use our own fears against us to achieve sales results. Our subconscious is learning and being brainwashed from a young age through visual media that most of us are not even aware of.

What sort of things do you do to stay mentally and physically healthy?
I love being active. I find it impossible to sit still for too long, unless I have a great book to read. I used to do heavy training — running, biking and the gym — but these days I prefer to do incidental exercise. I have a high cortisol level and a struggling adrenal system, so I was advised to do exercise that is more balancing. My high-stress, high-adrenaline job gives my heart enough of a workout! So I love to get out on my boat fishing and swimming, rowing and walking the dog along the sand. At home I walk a couple of miles every day and swim laps, usually in the ocean pool near my house. Every morning without fail I do a series of stretches and yoga in my shower and I'm always doing things around the house. I can haul a 154-pound anchor out of the water on my own and balance on the boat in any weather. I think these things are the most important as we age: *strength*, because you have to be able to get up and down, carry shopping and those kinds of things; *balance*, so you don't break any bones and end up in the hospital; and *flexibility*, because once you can't get your own shoes on or pull up your own undies and socks, they will pop you in a home.

'It's those little achievements that keep me going on hideous days and make me feel like I've had a win.'

▲

Your Health Is
Your Wealth

———

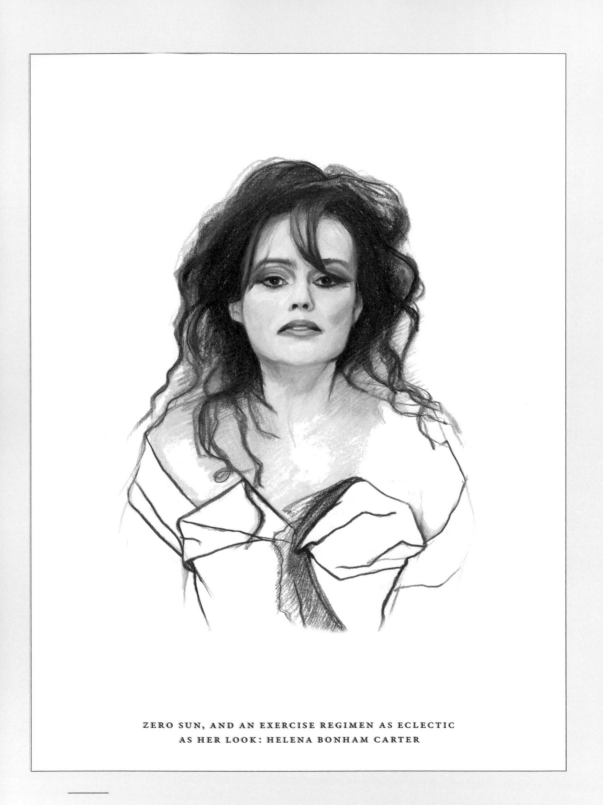

ZERO SUN, AND AN EXERCISE REGIMEN AS ECLECTIC
AS HER LOOK: HELENA BONHAM CARTER

That's my goal with my health, to stay as independent as possible, and die doing something I love, somewhere I want to be.

How do you deal with chronic pain, and what would be your advice for women living with it?
Fibromyalgia has been very challenging. I think of my pain in the third person most of the time — I don't know where I got that from, but it helps. I just think of it like a person who's trying to hold me back from whatever it is that I want to do, and almost challenge it: *Watch me do that thing you are trying to stop me from doing.* I give it a bit of attitude. When I'm flaring badly, there is not much I can do but wait it out and have lots of magnesium baths.

It's taught me a lot about myself and self-care. I'm much more aware of my physical health than ever before, because I got to the point where I couldn't hold a coffee cup or even get out of bed, and I had to go to the United States for treatment that wasn't available where I live. When you get to that stage and have lost the ability to push through mentally, it makes you reconsider everything about your lifestyle. I cut back on alcohol and late nights, increased my magnesium, iodine and chlorophyll intake dramatically, and took more sun without sunscreen to get my vitamin D levels up. I'm more aware of what I need to do daily to manage it, and I manage the pain and symptoms as much as I can with natural remedies and solutions first.

No matter how bad it is I get up, have a shower, stretch and walk my dog. I may then have to go back to bed, but it's those little achievements that keep me going on hideous days and make me feel like I've had a win.

How did you come to the decision to have a hysterectomy, and how are you feeling about your decision and recovery?
I had no choice about having a hysterectomy. I think that was the hardest to absorb. My GP and I were managing the fibromyalgia

Your Health Is
Your Wealth

and the symptoms cross over, so I had no idea there was anything wrong in that area until it became such acute pain in my midsection that it was obvious. I'd been having stomach upsets and bladder issues, but we tested for bugs as I travel a lot, and no infection was present in any tests of my bladder. No diabetes or anything even worth flagging. All my tests came back perfect every time. We thought it was just another fibromyalgia symptom.

I was in such incredible pain and bleeding so heavily that I got very scared. I asked my GP to send me for all the scans I could have of my abdominal and reproductive areas so we could finally get to the bottom of it. It wasn't livable pain — and I have a high tolerance for pain after years with fibro. I went to the radiologist that afternoon and she said I had to go to a gynecologist as soon as humanly possible because she could see seven or more tumors of various sizes that were about as big as oranges.

That was terrifying. I was so lucky that I have private health care and could get straight in to see a good gynecologist the following day. He broke the news in a very matter of fact way, which I appreciated. My womb was too damaged for any other alternative, and the fibroids were pressing on other internal organs, creating malfunctions and pain.

I still had to triple-check my options — I had been considering IVF, as my fertility (as far as my ovaries and hormones were concerned) was still in top shape. Devastatingly, three other gynecologists I consulted said the same thing. There was no way to save my womb, and I will never carry my own child. That's something I'm still working through; it's going to take some time to reconcile, I think. It was such a rush from diagnosis to operation. The test results came back and the tumors were benign fibroids.

Recovery is annoying, slow and mind-numbingly boring. My emotions are all over the place, I'm bursting into tears randomly as the finality of it hits me in waves. Work helps take my mind off it and I'm still getting up and doing as much as I can every day. I'll be okay, it could have been way worse. I've since read stories about women who have gone through the same thing, except their tumors were malignant. I've also just lost a friend to ovarian cancer.

So really, I'm thankful. It's affirming my love of life, and I want to live the biggest one possible.

Reaching out for help from those around you is a sign of strength—we all need our tribe.

Your Health Is
Your Wealth

FOCUS ON JOY

▲

Even with the best health and self-care intentions, life sometimes throws us a curveball. When a partner or child falls ill, the last thing we often feel able to do is look after ourselves, but that's when it should take precedence above all else.

To survive the tough times, take care of yourself by applying all the basics mentioned earlier, and feel free to add in some nutrition supplements such as magnesium for stress and helping with better sleep. Take regular breaks for yourself — a walk around the park, a quick swim, or a 30-minute nap to recharge — and lean on help from a 'back-up': your partner, child or a friend you can trust. Find at least one other person you can speak to, even if it's a paid professional. You need to be able to share what you're going through, as bottling it up will only lead to anxiety and health issues.

Stay present. Don't let the fear take over, and find joy in the small things, like a beautiful sunrise, children laughing or a nourishing meal with friends.

Try to remember, life can be good, even when it's not.

The
Power Age

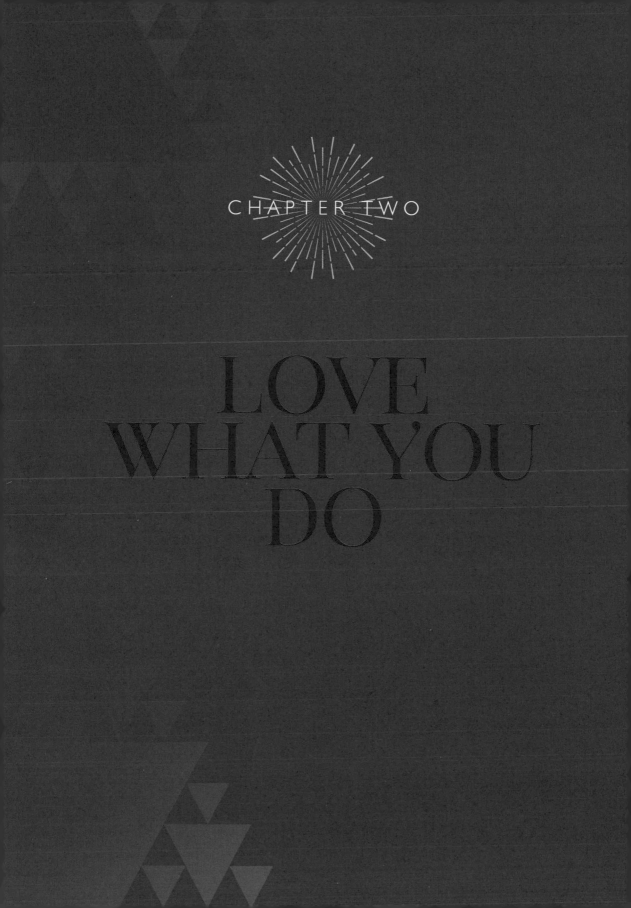

CHAPTER TWO

LOVE
WHAT YOU
DO

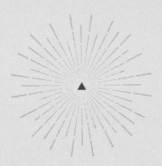

The well-worn adage 'Love what you do and you'll never work a day in your life' has thoroughly pervaded the modern idea of what we demand and expect for ourselves in terms of our productive lives. Fair enough. Many of us spend a huge portion of our waking hours at work (often more than we spend with family or friends), so it seems important that we enjoy what we do each day as much as humanly possible. The same holds true in later life — perhaps even more so than it did when we were younger or still figuring ourselves out, and the need to make every day count wasn't quite so pressing.

As Anu Partanen aptly puts it in her book, *The Nordic Theory of Everything: In search of a better life*, 'a woman is meant to be more than a caretaker for her man and children. She ought to have her own purpose, her own will, her own career, including her own salary.' Economic independence, no matter what age we are, is such an important key to self-confidence. Conversely, feeling unhappy or devoid of choice when it comes to our work lives can be intensely undermining to our sense of self.

Whether you're in a senior career position or not, midlife is a great time to pause, take stock, check in with where you are and where you want to be, and how you hope the next years of your life will roll out. Because now is the time to change it up if you'd like to — there is no better opportunity.

If your job is making you miserable, consider what you can do about it. An element of work is about putting food on the table, but nothing is worth risking your health and sanity for. Don't stay in a toxic or unpleasant work environment if you can help it; this will wreak havoc on your life over time. It might feel like the options open to us career-wise narrow as we age, but experience will always be valued in a knowledge-based economy, and this is the way of the future.

As an article by Jessica Bennett in *The New York Times* reported in 2019, there are more women over the age of fifty in the United States today than at any other point in history, and the news has been filled with influential women over sixty in recent times: 'It seems that older women, long invisible or shunted aside, are experiencing an unfamiliar sensation: power,' she wrote. Nancy Pelosi (the 78-year-old who was reelected to the U.S. House of Representatives), Glenn Close (who bested four younger women to win a Golden Globe for her role in the film adaptation of Meg Wolitzer's book *The Wife*) and Susan Zirinsky (who took over at CBS News at the age of 66), were just a few of the women mentioned. According to data from the U.S. Census Bureau, women in this age bracket are healthier, working longer, and have more income than previous generations, which is 'creating modest but real progress in their visibility and stature'. This statistic is echoed in other Western nations.

Of course, men have been holding the top jobs well into their seventh, eighth and even ninth decades for generations, but take heart: change is afoot. You have a right to be here, and you have something unique to offer the world. Really focus on what that is and remember: *anything is possible*.

Love What
You Do

Savour the moment

Many people in their forties or older have reached senior positions, or at least have the confidence that comes from decades of experience in their chosen field. Any good employer will agree that women of this age are such an asset in the workplace — they've been around a while, know how things work, and have a wealth of experience and knowledge to offer. If they've also juggled busy careers with caring for family, they know how to manage their time and priorities.

Make the most of this situation by being the sort of woman others will look up to or want to be mentored by. Extend a helping hand to those who ask or seem to need it, and leave the schoolyard far behind in regards to petty rivalries.

This is your time. A time to stand in your strength, work hard, stay focused and shine bright.

Do a career inventory

If you're stuck in a rut, examine your options. What is it you've always dreamed of doing? Is it cutting hair, working in events management, or making a difference through charitable works? Would you like to work outside an office for a change, or pursue a more creative path — did you always see yourself as a writer or an artist, perhaps? Do you want to be in a boardroom, influencing how corporate structures or government work? Set about making it happen.

Maybe you need to take on a new course of study to develop your skills? Put yourself out there. Apply for courses of study or different roles (it's staggering how many people seem desperately unhappy in their jobs, but don't take this first, crucial step), and weigh up how important it is to you against the temporary loss of income — particularly if you have to take a break from paid work to study.

If money's an issue (rarely is it not), work towards your goal by squirrelling away funds for a less lucrative period while you change direction. Or aim high and set your sights on a role that pays what you are worth. To gain the confidence to make that leap, search out

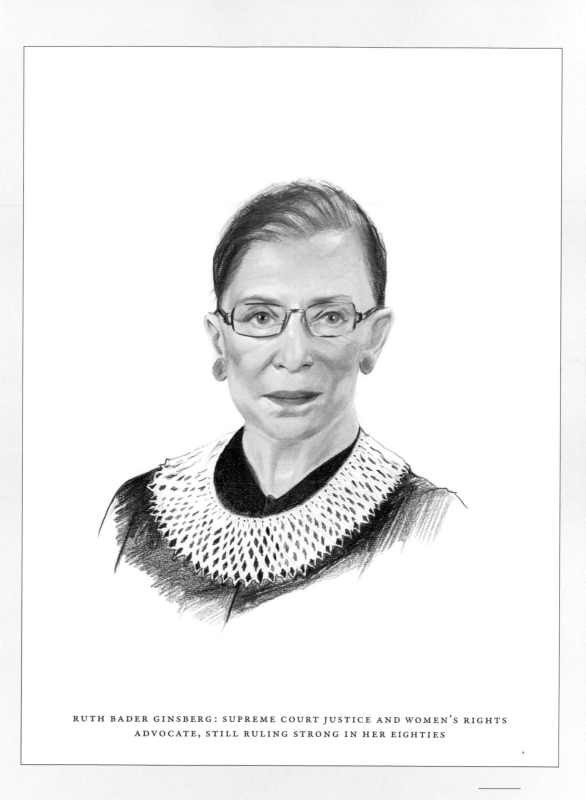

RUTH BADER GINSBERG: SUPREME COURT JUSTICE AND WOMEN'S RIGHTS
ADVOCATE, STILL RULING STRONG IN HER EIGHTIES

a human resources manager or career consultant, or a female role model who is already in their dream job, to help you gain clarity.

Hit refresh

There's always an option that doesn't include chucking out the baby with the bathwater: rediscover your love for what you already do. In practical terms, perhaps this means making a conscious effort to disengage yourself from noxious office politics, or joining women's networks in your industry that can help you forge new contacts and move sideways, or into a new role in a new organisation. What first drew you to your work, and do the same fundamentals still hold true? Could you start working for yourself in the same industry, by setting up your own business?

Often all it takes is a shift in perspective to see that the negatives as we perceive them are, in fact, positives. We're here to learn, after all, and it can be amazingly transformative to see things with fresh eyes.

Perfect the pivot

A career pivot, at any age, is different to a regular job search. If you don't have experience in a new field, be prepared to overcome questions from any potential employer about why you're making the change, and construct a coherent career story to explain your rationale for making the switch. Make sure it is clear and believable.

Bring potential employers along for the ride with an engaging story that makes it obvious you're not just testing the waters or casting about because you're bored. Proof of your determination and intention will help, such as a diploma in a new course of relevant study, or letters of recommendation from people with experience in the same area. Seek membership in career-appropriate organisations.

Don't be defensive about your reasons for making a career move, and don't emphasise your newness to the role. Rather, highlight your relevant experience: draw parallels between your current expertise and the expertise you'll need to exhibit in your new role.

Ditch the romance

For some, the idea of *loving* what you do is often equated with success at making a *living* out of it. But one of the side effects of monetising something you adore can also mean that it no longer brings you joy. It can also create a huge amount of pressure.

Elizabeth Gilbert's book *Big Magic: Creative living beyond fear* questions the popular idea of following your passion so exclusively. As she explains, 'I've seen artists drive themselves broke and crazy because of this insistence that they are not legitimate creators unless they can exclusively live off their creativity.'

Even when art does pay the bills, it changes your dynamic with it. As Gilbert says in *Big Magic*, following your passion can be an 'unhelpful and even cruel suggestion at times ... a lot of people don't know exactly what their passion is, or they may have multiple passions, or they may go through a midlife change of passion — all of which can leave them feeling confused and blocked and insecure.'

The point is, don't romanticise the creative path. Love what you do, but don't insist that your work be creatively fulfilling *all* the time. Even successful artists find work just that, sometimes: *work*. More to the point, examine whether your job is meaningful. It takes a load of determination and effort to succeed on a creative path — just as much (if not more) than in other fields. Don't valorize it. Many 'successful' endeavours require creativity, too, such as science, for example. It's just a matter of perception.

And always remember that creativity can be fulfilled in so many other ways. Explore creative hobbies and extracurricular pursuits that feed your soul, and find a balance that makes you happy. There's nothing wrong with being a passionate amateur or enthusiast — and you may even find that this can open doors in later life during your so-called 'retirement'.

Love What
You Do

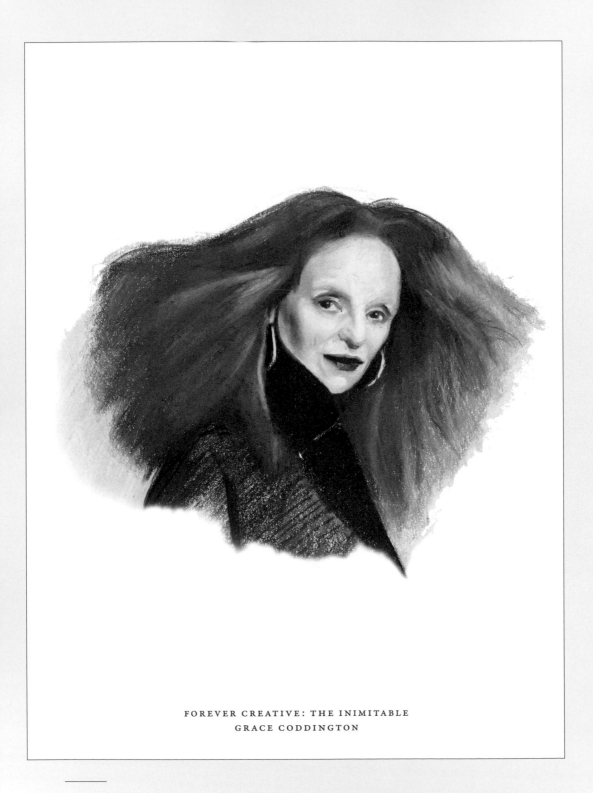

FOREVER CREATIVE: THE INIMITABLE
GRACE CODDINGTON

It's never too late to seek out a mentor

Q&A WITH DR. KIRSTIN FERGUSON, BUSINESS LEADER AND INDEPENDENT COMPANY DIRECTOR

▲

Dr. Kirstin Ferguson, 46, is an Adjunct Professor at the Queensland University of Technology Business School and sits on private and government boards. She is the creator of the global social media campaign #CelebratingWomen, and co-author of *Women Kind: Unlocking the power of women supporting women*.

What do you think women can gain from effective mentoring?
Women who are prepared to seek out a mentor, listen and learn from them and then become mentors to *other* women will find themselves part of the shared, collective power that comes from women supporting women. Mentoring forms a very important part of that power.

All women benefit from being mentored, since it opens your mind to thinking about problems and ways of considering the world in a new way. It often exposes women to leaders from new industries or sectors, which also expands the unique ways of approaching an issue.

It is also an important period of time carved out of what is

Love What
You Do

otherwise often a busy working day to focus solely on the mentee — their aspirations, personal development and challenges. This time is precious and when well used, it is also invaluable for the professional and personal development of women.

When would you suggest looking for a mentor — and where is a good place to start?
It is never too late to seek out a mentor, as we can all benefit from mentors throughout our lives. I have a 'buffet' of mentors that I call upon for different reasons depending on the advice I may be seeking help with. I have had some of my mentors for more than 20 years and continue to seek their wisdom and counsel as needed.

Most of my mentors have been found 'organically' — that is, through informal networks, whether with direct work colleagues or others within my business network. I have also had mentors who have been matched with me through formal networks, and those mentoring relationships have tended to continue long after the formal aspect of the connection has ended.

You might find your mentors in the most unexpected places, so always be open to listening respectfully to different points of view, and to those people who are willing to invest time and energy into seeing you do well.

How should you prepare for your first meeting with a mentor, what are some goals you could be setting — and how many sessions would you suggest having together?
A new mentee should always come very well prepared to every meeting with their mentor.

At the first meeting, it is important to make clear to your new mentor that you value their time, and to come to that meeting with a clear set of goals you have for the sessions. You should also have done a lot of research on your new mentor to understand their career history, so you know specifically what experience you might

'All women benefit from being mentored, since it opens your mind to thinking about problems and ways of considering the world in a new way.'

▲

be hoping to draw upon.

Some goals you might like to consider could be around how to progress within your organisation or industry, how to become a more effective leader, understanding what training or courses may benefit you, or seeking advice on specific challenges you may be grappling with.

Formal mentoring sessions are ideally held every one or two months, and will continue as long as you and your mentor feel they are valuable.

Informal mentoring can last a lifetime.

Are there any clear boundaries that should be set, and what would they be?
One of the more disappointing messages to emerge after the #MeToo movement were comments from men (and sometimes also women) suggesting men would no longer be able to mentor a woman. I think that would be a really unfortunate development, because we know that women benefit from being able to be mentored by those in senior positions, with influence and power, who so often continue to be men.

Boundaries in any mentoring relationship will be based on common sense. This will be a professional relationship, and so the way you conduct yourself in your professional environment should extend to any mentoring relationship.

I don't think mentors are necessarily there to work through your personal problems; however, a good mentor will also know just enough to realize that if you are struggling with a personal issue, this is likely to impact your professional day.

Ultimately, being in a mentor / mentee relationship requires candor, honesty and vulnerability — and common sense will always help determine the appropriate boundaries.

Love What
You Do

Mastering the art of reinvention

INTERVIEW WITH KIRSTEN GALLIOTT,
SENIOR MEDIA EXECUTIVE

▲

With over 25 years' experience in newspapers, magazines, television and radio, Kirsten Galliott, 49, has had several jobs at the helm over the course of her career, including Editor of *InStyle* magazine. She now manages three in-house titles at a major airline, overseeing more than sixty staff. We spoke about what it takes to ride the waves of change.

In an industry beset by constant challenges during the digital age, Kirsten has managed to succeed by staying one step ahead, moving from one high-profile position to the next and reinventing herself at each stage.

'I don't believe in doing something without doing it well. I'm also quite good at knowing when to go,' Kirsten explains. In discussions with a previous employer about a journalism role, she was told she had to be prepared for 'churnalism' (quick, under-researched writing for online platforms) — but found the idea of it so abhorrent, she knew she couldn't stay. 'Just because you're writing for digital doesn't mean it can't be of a high quality,' she says.

Kirsten has always followed her intuition and thought laterally about the next step in her career. 'In this age, people

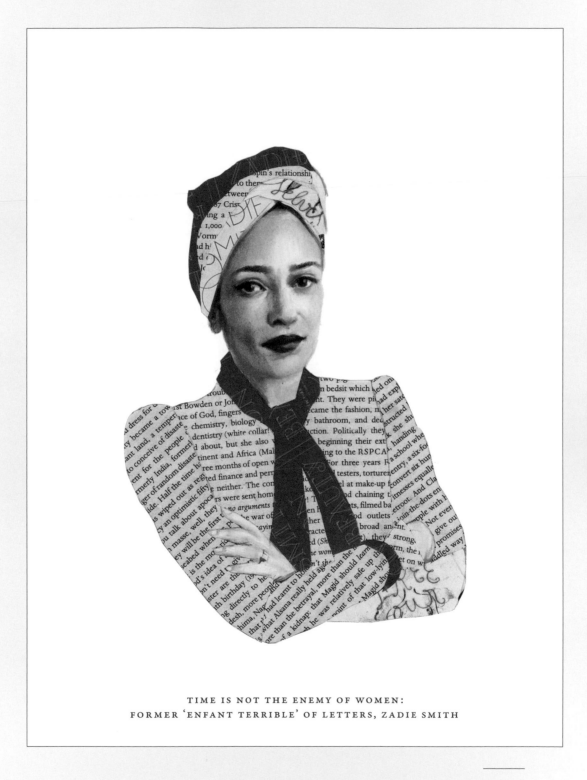

TIME IS NOT THE ENEMY OF WOMEN:
FORMER 'ENFANT TERRIBLE' OF LETTERS, ZADIE SMITH

have so many different jobs. You have to keep up if you want a career with longevity. I've had to be prepared to learn in every new job I've had.'

Many women find the biggest challenge is reinventing themselves after having children, or finding a way to work that balances the demands of home life and a busy career; ageing parents and health issues can all take their toll.

'I do think it's our responsibility to lift other women up,' says Kirsten. 'In terms of hiring women with children, there's always going to be a slight thing in your head that says it'll be so much easier to hire someone who's available 24/7, but that's a very dangerous assumption to make. Selfishly, you want someone who's going to dedicate themselves to the role. When I was working as editor of *InStyle* magazine, I had that moment. But I interviewed someone at the time who had a roster of working mothers. She told me it was hard to manage, but worth it because they are so dedicated and hardworking. Everything she said really resonated with me. I ended up hiring a deputy editor with three children who also came to work with me in the next position I took on.

'There will be times that working mothers will have to duck off to school assemblies or whatever it is — and I'm one of those mothers as well — but we just need to make sure that we're giving our other staff without families the same flexibility that working mothers are being given. It can be a logistical nightmare, but it's worth it.'

The main breadwinner in her family, Kirsten is 49 but expects to work for at least another fifteen years. 'I was 38 when I had my first daughter, and 41 when I had my second. I loved having my children later, because I feel like they keep me young. The only challenge is having a very demanding career, and making sure I have enough time for them. It's always a mad juggle.'

'In this age, people have so many different jobs. I've had to be prepared to learn in every new job I've had.'

▲

The
Power Age

Be an agent for change

INTERVIEW WITH CRIS PARKER, THEATRE COMPANY
FOUNDER TURNED BUSINESSWOMAN

▲

Having switched from a life in the theatre to a successful corporate career, Cris Parker, 54, understands the career pivot well. She is now a senior businesswoman at The Banking & Finance Oath, an industry-led initiative that helps financial organisations operate ethically. Here we look at how curiosity and desire for change can engender change.

'I never had a vision for what my life would look like, or what career path I would take,' Cris explains. 'Exploring ideas I find interesting and challenging has driven my journey.

'I fell into storytelling at an early age, co-founding a theatre company in New York City. I've also been a filmmaker and lived a lot of life in between. After obtaining a psychology degree, I started working at The Ethics Centre and was offered the role of Executive at The Banking and Finance Oath. I love a challenge and really enjoy working with people.

'The corporate world has a way of dehumanising, particularly through language, but also through the idea that what matters is what can be measured. In my role I started to talk to people and they cared, they were smart, and they wanted to have a positive impact. I enjoy working in an area that helps encourage the kind of behaviour

Love What
You Do

55

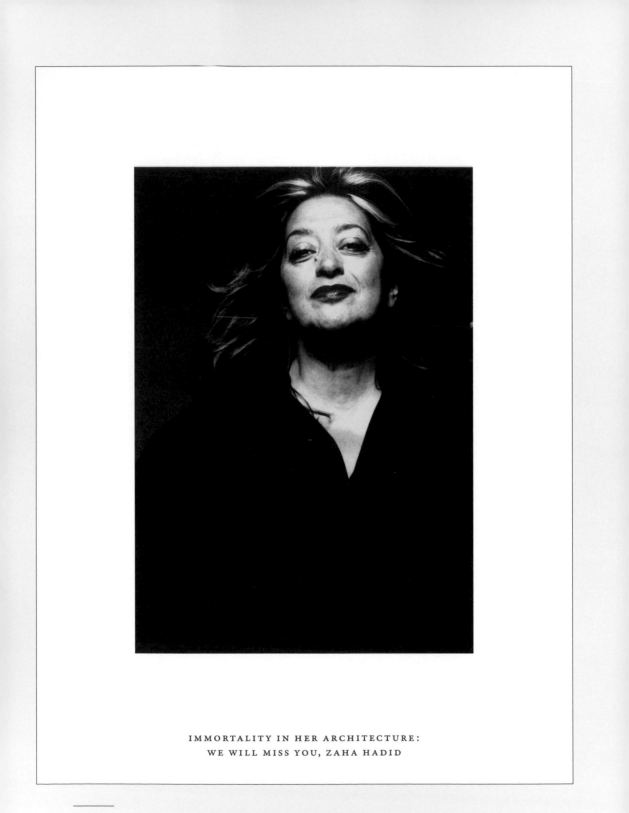

IMMORTALITY IN HER ARCHITECTURE:
WE WILL MISS YOU, ZAHA HADID

and practices that support the sort of society we want to see.'

Her advice to women wishing to succeed in business or corporate environments is to own it.

'Surround yourself with like-minded people — and, most importantly, take other women with you. Be mindful that making "tough" or hard decisions doesn't make you too self-focused. I've seen people change because they were not willing to be vulnerable with their colleagues, not even for a second.'

In regards to the issues facing women, things are changing in the corporate world — but not fast enough, says Cris.

'There are so many smart, fabulous older women in financial services who are respected and who lead the way well, but ageism definitely exists. Sexism is a little different. It's more a lack of inclusion; how many women are willing to blow off work for an afternoon and have a late lunch with their male colleagues? Are they even invited? Many women need to use every second of their working hours to get the job done, because their home life starts on the way home.'

The hardest and most deplorable thing women deal with in the work force is the pay gap, Cris says. 'What is measured matters, and in business that is with money. This message is simply unacceptable.'

'Surround yourself with like-minded people — and, most importantly, take other women with you.'

▲

Dealing with ageism

If you think you're the recipient of discriminatory behaviour, call it out with your human resources department. If you work in a small company or non-corporate environment, you could try handling it yourself with your manager or the owner of the business, to help bring the issue out into the open. In today's climate, no company wants to be disgraced publicly, so you should politely, but firmly, put your point across and ask for it to be addressed. If you face difficulties, you can always escalate it to a higher authority, such as the Equal Employment Opportunity Commission.

Love What
You Do

The possibilities are endless

Q&A WITH WENDY HARMER
AUTHOR, JOURNALIST AND COMEDIAN

▲

Wendy Harmer, 64, is known for her work as a comedian in television and on radio, and as a bestselling author of comic novels and children's fiction. Here she reflects on her rich and multifaceted career.

When did you realise you first wanted to work in comedy, and what sort of change did it require from what you were currently doing?

In the mid-80s I was working as a political journalist with *The Sun-News Pictorial* newspaper and was asked to write a feature story on the so-called 'New Wave' of comedy. It was fate. The night of stand-up, satire and song was amazing, brilliant, I adored it! I knew instantly that I wanted to be up on that stage, too.

Mere months later (and to the astonishment of the newsroom), I quit my job and took another at the *Melbourne Times*, where I could report on state politics three days a week, working on my stand-up routines and performing at night. It was an exhausting time, as I worked into the wee hours in the comedy clubs and in the newsroom by day, but was finally able to go into full-time entertaining when I was hired to be in a children's program on ABC. My first real hosting job on *The Big Gig* came not long after.

The
Power Age

To make a living in showbiz and support my family all these years has been my greatest achievement. I still can't believe that leap of faith paid off for me.

How have some of your roles challenged you?
For the eleven years I spent in breakfast radio on 2Day FM, I knew what time it was, almost to the minute. Getting up so early, giving birth to my two children along the way, juggling social engagements and still performing shows now and then meant every moment was so precious. I got up at 3.30 am to breastfeed and use the breast pump for more feeds. I took my son to the U.S. to broadcast for the Oscars when he was only three months old. What was I thinking?! Thank goodness for my dedicated house husband, Brendan, who was utterly supportive through all the madness. Looking back, I feel like I was jet-lagged for an entire decade.

These days I'm back on the breakfast shift with ABC Radio and up at 3.45 am, and again, my husband is with me every step of the way. At least these days, it's without two squirming bodies between us in the king-sized bed, and the house renovations are finished. As I make the long drive from our home in the Northern Beaches to work, I wonder if I've seen more sunrises over the Harbour Bridge than anyone else. That's a blessing I never take for granted.

What were some of the catalysts for you moving into different fields, such as writing children's books, for example? Were you concerned at any point about leaving certain roles behind to reinvent yourself?
I've never seen my career in terms of purposeful reinvention, but rather a change in gear or shift in emphasis. The areas I've worked in — stage, TV, newspaper columns, books, broadcasting, plays and online media — all exploit my twin talents with the

Love What
You Do

written and spoken word. I see that thread in everything I have done or attempted to do. And I've usually done a few things simultaneously — like write a book while I'm performing, or a play when I'm broadcasting. And I've always had a column to write for some 20 years or so.

Everything seems to feed, quite naturally, into the next thing (but I've never tried to dance in public — I know my limits!). I'm not one to rely on any one project coming to fruition, and usually have lots of things happening all at once.

Sometimes a break in proceedings can be the catalyst — a year on 'gardening leave' from 2Day FM after my contract was terminated early gave me the clear air I needed to write my novels and kids' books.

There's never a shortage of things to do and my mantra is: *Life is short — try to make every mistake possible!*

How have you dealt with fallow periods in your career?
I can't recall ever having a 'fallow' time. I have always had a strong creative drive, a capacity for hard work, and an ability to look at things differently. I'm usually brimming with plans for the next project.

There's a couple of reasons for why this might be. As a journalist, you're always seeking to learn the mechanisms for how things work. You read widely, take in a lot of information and look at everything with a skeptical eye. Comedy teaches you how to make oblique connections with the information you gather, and see things as an outsider does.

When you take that step back, think and observe, you can often see patterns emerging ... What's missing, and what's just around the corner? Rest assured though, my bottom drawer of projects stamped 'Fail' is just as full as the top one.

'I've never seen my career in terms of purposeful reinvention, but rather a change in gear or shift in emphasis.'

▲

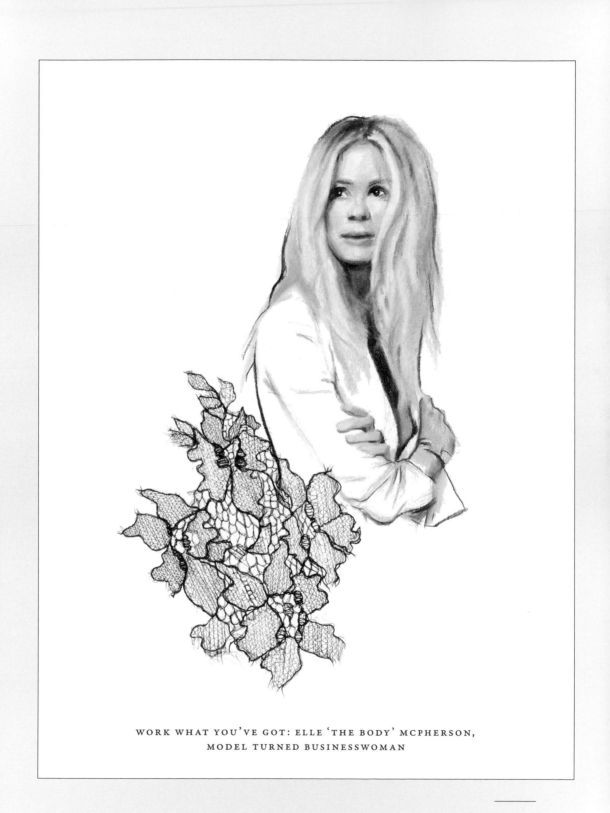

WORK WHAT YOU'VE GOT: ELLE 'THE BODY' MCPHERSON,
MODEL TURNED BUSINESSWOMAN

What advice would you give to women who maybe feel stuck or like they're not following the career that best suits them?
Know your limits. What are you willing to risk financially? What are you really good at? How hard are you willing to work? That's the stuff everyone tells you, right?

But beyond that are the possibilities, and they are endless. So maybe take a jump into the wild blue yonder and follow your Girls' Own adventure. *We're only going around once* is my other mantra. I've always had a back-up plan to be a salsa mogul. 'Wendy's Hot and Sultry Salsa' ... you'd buy that, right?

Wendy's top tips for a fulfilling career

- Don't wait for the phone to ring. Ring first!
- Have plans marked A, B, C and D — and be in love with plan E, too.
- Find a willing accomplice in your life's plan, but don't tell them everything you're thinking of. Surprise them!
- Don't always expect a career to be fulfilling. It may actually be that other thing you do that's the most rewarding.
- Always remember that life is what happens when you're making other plans. Everyone thinks John Lennon said that, but he didn't — so if you understand that you'll always be misquoted, you'll have a happier life.

* **Bonus tip:** Do. Not. Even. Think. Of. Looking. Up. Your. Images. On. The. Internet. Ever.

If you plunge into the unknown,
you're not going to hit the bottom

Q&A WITH SALLY LOANE, JOURNALIST, BROADCASTER
AND CEO OF THE FINANCIAL SERVICES COUNCIL

▲

After 25 years as a journalist, Sally Loane, 62, switched to the
corporate sector, and is now head of the Financial Services Council.
Here she reflects on what it takes to carve out a new pathway.

**You've had such a diverse career. What would you say to women
who've been out of the workforce while raising children, or are
considering a big career change to follow a different path?**
One of the most difficult things you can do in life is shift direction
— whether it's returning to work after having children, or changing
not just jobs, but entire careers.

A friend said something kind that has stayed with me over
decades of diverse work challenges: 'Don't worry, you'll be fine.
This is like bungy jumping. It will feel like you're going over a cliff,
but you have a great big piece of elastic rope around your ankles
which will break your fall and bounce you back up.'

I've kept that advice in mind every time I've faced a new
challenge in the three very different careers I've had since I started
work as a journalism cadet at 22.

After 25 years as a journalist working in print, television and
radio, I switched from journalism to work in the corporate sector.

Love What
You Do

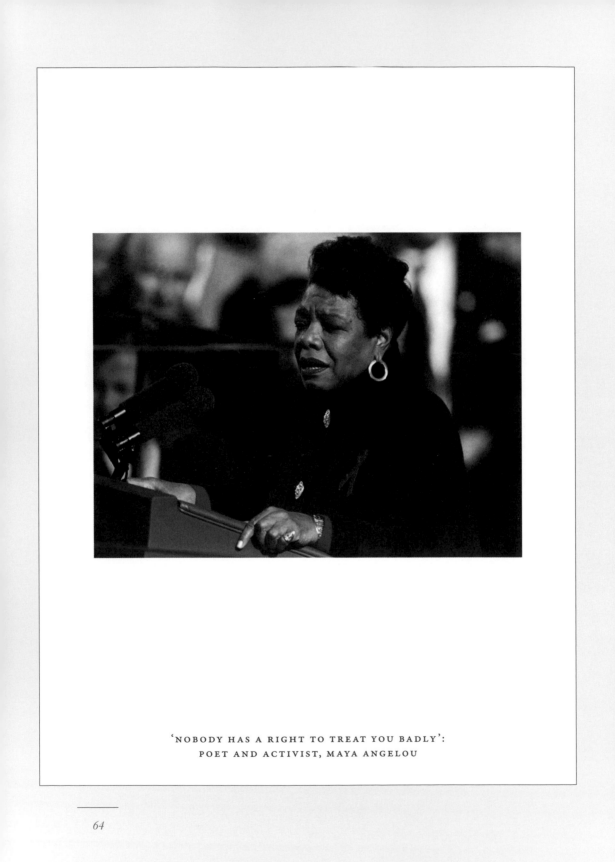

'NOBODY HAS A RIGHT TO TREAT YOU BADLY':
POET AND ACTIVIST, MAYA ANGELOU

My next move after nine years of working for Coca-Cola Amatil was to lead a peak industry organisation, the Financial Services Council, representing more than 100 firms across superannuation funds, life insurances, advice licensees, trustees and fund managers. This was my first CEO role, and again, I faced another steep learning curve in a whole new sector.

If you want to switch careers as dramatically as I have, it helps to like challenges. It's said that women are not always as brashly confident as men and suffer from 'imposter syndrome', but I'm not sure it's that clear cut. I think many of us are innately cautious and it's ingrained in some of us to strive for perfection. This can hold us back. If you want to venture outside your comfort zone, remember there's a magic elastic rope on your leg, and if you plunge into the unknown, you're not going to hit the bottom.

'If you want to switch careers as dramatically as I have, it helps to like challenges.'

▲

What are your thoughts on the #MeToo movement and modern female empowerment?
I often find myself thinking about the young women who are facing very challenging times through no fault of their own because they've spoken up about sexual harassment. Every generation of women since time began has endured this, but the difference is that this generation of women has the legal means to do something about it. My generation actually made the laws our daughters are using, and I could not be more glad — even though the consequences for utilising those laws are sometimes harrowing.

Social media has a lot to answer for. It's not only created cover for the most craven cowards to abuse and harass women and girls, it's exacerbated a general shift towards the extreme polarisation of debates. By all means, support causes you believe in, like #MeToo, but beware of getting sucked into a black echo chamber. Social media is a bit like talkback radio — it's never a measure of what people think — it only represents the screechiest, and often loopiest, of squeaky wheels.

Love What
You Do

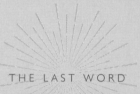

THE LAST WORD

FOLLOW YOUR TRUE CALLING

▲

▸ **With change the only constant,** approaching our work with a lightness and curiosity allows us to seize opportunities when they manifest. Remember, every challenge is an opportunity for growth.

▸ **Stay in your own lane.** Ignore what others are up to and avoid 'the comparison trap'. Follow the path that's right for you and you alone, looking to others only for inspiration in general.

▸ **Push for parity** with men, and for being paid what you're worth. Don't 'put up and shut up'. When negotiating for a higher salary, do your research. Look at comparative roles within your industry and provide your employer with good, solid evidence to explain why you're worth that amount. If a man is being paid one salary and you have commensurate experience, there is no reason why you should be paid less. Do remember that timing is also key: ask when the pay raises for the year ahead are considered, and set up a formal meeting (in writing) beforehand.

▸ **Trust your gut.** You know that niggling feeling that something's not right? Heed it. Work out what your calling is and make a change for the better. Career satisfaction awaits — or, at the very least, your next adventure.

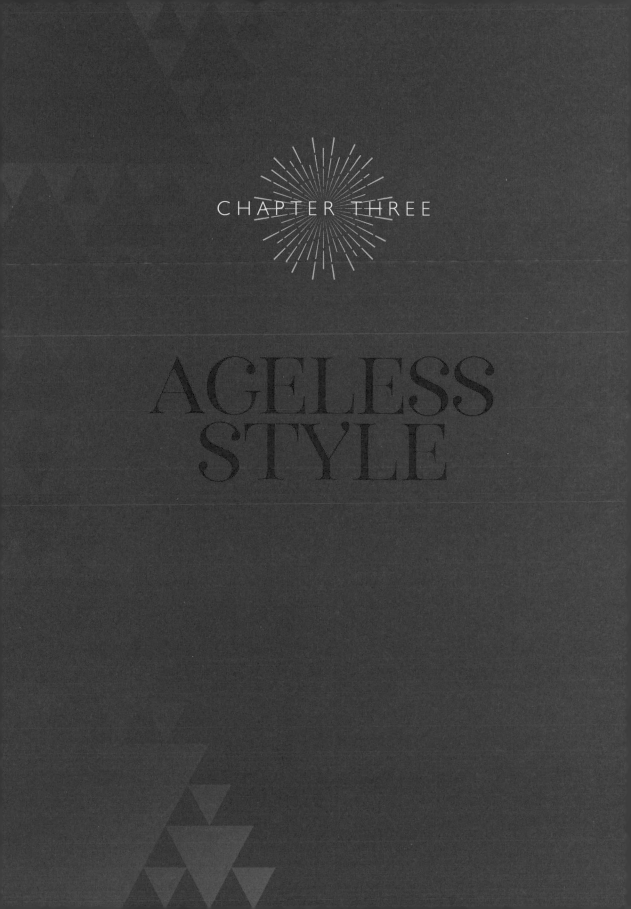

CHAPTER THREE

AGELESS STYLE

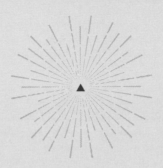

As legendary Hollywood costume designer Edith Head once said, 'You can have anything you want in life if you dress for it.' And as fashion designer Dame Vivienne Westwood, 78, herself observed, you'll enjoy a more interesting life if you wear impressive clothes. Amen to that.

There really is something magnificent about a woman who knows her style and wears it with confidence. True style transcends age, class, racial and gender barriers — it's the way you walk, the way you hold yourself and the conviction with which you present yourself every day, almost regardless of how you dress. But there are ways to create an air about you and project to the world who you are in an instant without uttering a single word, and one important way is through your clothing.

Fashion is not the frivolity it's often made out to be. It's a reflection of who we are and the message we wish to project to the world. By god though, it can be fun!

While our teens and twenties are all about experimenting and trying on a whole range of different identities for size, it's usually in our thirties when most of us find our feet style-wise. The trick is not to stick with your best discoveries religiously, but to continue to grow and evolve over the years as the trends change and you mature. You want your clothes to take the fabulous person within — the adventures you've been on, the wisdom you've gained — and share it with the world at large.

The fashion industry is awash with older women projecting great style, and now more than ever. Look to them for inspiration. Remember that great Karen Walker eyewear campaign using older models? Genius. And the recent catwalk show in Milan featuring the original supermodels — Naomi Campbell, Christy Turlington, Cindy Crawford, Helena Christensen and Claudia Schiffer — all in their late forties and early fifties, who turned out in jaw-dropping form to steal the show? But you don't need the genes of a supermodel. You don't even need to be beautiful.

All you need is that special something, that secret ingredient, that *je ne sais quoi*: style. And here's how to get it.

Forget age-appropriate dressing

Throw out the rule book — there isn't anything a woman *can't* or *shouldn't* wear after a certain age. If you have the legs for it, a miniskirt can look fabulous forever. Consider Italian fashion journalist Anna Dello Russo, 57, who has become famous for her flamboyant style and risqué hemlines. Or Carine Roitfeld, 67, former editor of French *Vogue*, who wears minis, vampy black lace *and* leopard print without looking like the punchline of a joke. Whether you like their taste is neither here nor there — each of these women owns it. You can rock hair plaits with panache in your nineties, or strut streetwear in your sixties, but these are just some of the trends we're told should 'never be seen' on an older woman. Boo to that.

Chutzpah can carry you a hell of a long way. Whatever it is that floats your boat, just go for it.

Ageless
Style

69

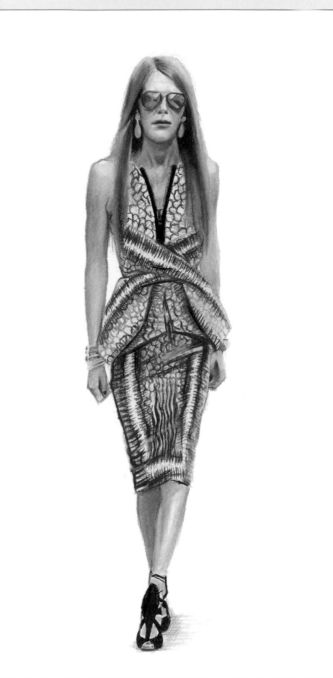

THE QUEEN OF FLAMBOYANT HIGH FASHION, ANNA DELLO RUSSO
BREAKS ALL THE 'RULES', YET ALWAYS LOOKS FANTASTIC

Find your own staples

There are various schools of thought: French fashion icon Inès de La Fressange is all in favour of simple classics and man-style dressing in shirts, blazers and brogues. And Parisian women do look effortlessly chic. But what if you don't have the figure for those so-called staple items? Or if simple shapes and styles bore you to tears?

Find out what suits you. Find the colours and prints and cuts that work for you, and never stop experimenting. What flatters you most, and what makes you feel confident or the best version of yourself? That's what you're aiming for. This will change. Roll with it.

Consider where your eye is drawn and why. What makes your heart skip a beat? Think about your fashion background — the era you grew up in, the things that influenced you. Was it a favourite overseas trip where you were charmed by a place's style signature, perhaps, or a movement like punk, which Vivienne Westwood still continues to draw on in her late seventies? Or do you like the straight-up classics with a twist? Amp it up. Be yourself. As Oscar Wilde said, everybody else is already taken.

If you feel confused about what's 'you', try buying some fashion magazines and dog-earing the pages that catch your eye. When you're done, turn to the front, go through those images that spoke to you most, and analyse *why*. Do you tend to gravitate towards a bold palette, or is monochrome more your thing? Do you like 1940s-inspired crisp dressing and shapes, or are you more of a hippie '60s or '70s chick who hates feeling buttoned-up and straight-laced?

Go high–low

As our wardrobes (and bank balances, hopefully) grow, and we learn what suits us more and more, it's vital not to get stuck in a rut and keep going back to the same familiar items again and again. Or constantly be buying 'up'. Being stuck in a fashion time warp is ageing, but so is wearing head-to-toe designer clothing — at least when it's obvious that you're doing so. Blatant labels are out (unless it's in the form of hip streetwear), and who wants to be a walking advertisement, anyway? So-called luxury brands are not the status symbols they once were. Quality, yes. Labels, no. Or only when worn in moderation.

A far better way to look fresh, relevant and on-trend (dare I say, *young*) is to adopt a high–low attitude. This means a mix of special, classic or designer pieces; something fun and stylish; and a vintage item or two — either pulled from your own wardrobe or found in a market or thrift shop.

Tips on tear sheets

▸ The best way to identify your style is to collect real or virtual 'tear sheets'. These are pictures from fashion magazines which feature favourite outfits or pieces. When you compile them over a number of years, it becomes apparent what you do and don't like.

▸ Pin pictures up inside your wardrobe door at the beginning of a new season, and look to them when you're feeling *meh*. It's a great form of inspiration to pull together a sharp outfit for the day.

▸ The internet is awash with millions of images you can draw from for your own style inspiration. How about setting up a Pinterest page specifically for compiling your own ideas? Or keeping a few pages open on your browser, just to remind you?

▸ Take a leaf out of your favourite celebrities' books, or those who have roughly the same body shape or haircut as you. These women will have spent thousands on expert styling advice over the years. Crib from them, and consider why their outfits or style seem to work so well.

There are certain brands to favour and continue to wear for years. Sure, some of these are placed at the pricier end of the spectrum — save for purchases that are worth calculating at a cost-per-wear sum on for decades, such as the Chanel 2.55 (a classic evening bag Coco Chanel named after the month she created it, February 1955), which will never go out of style.

But you don't always need to go high-end. Sometimes there's nothing more fun than finding a vintage or second-hand item to add a little zing to your wardrobe and instantly update your look. Or a streetwear purchase that feels cool, fun and up-to-date — as long as you'll wear it more than once. Fast fashion is a planet killer.

Great pieces for the ageless wardrobe

▸ White linen T-shirts, white structured cotton shirts, or creamy silk blouses, depending on your shape and style preference, for work or home

▸ Structured or loose blazers

▸ Well-tailored black separates

▸ A 'little' black dress (really just a well-made go-to frock, but black is timeless and goes with almost everything)

▸ Denim separates — jackets, skirts, wide-legged jeans … the list is endless

▸ A touch of dramatic animal print, either in a shirt, skirt, shoes, handbag or scarf … or, if you're feeling adventurous, a jumpsuit or full-length frock for a night on the town

▸ Slides or sandals in summer

▸ A red lip

▸ Dark sunglasses

▸ Great leather brogues — if you're feeling flush, plump for handmade

Be your wardrobe's bouncer

Have a strictly one-in, one-out policy — it's going to be so much easier to keep your wardrobe under control and find an easy outfit for the day if you do. Some women know how many pieces they have, down to the number, and cull every time they find something new. It's a clever idea.

Do an inventory today. Make a list of missing items, such as that perfect black long-sleeved top you'll wear so often throughout winter underneath dresses, jackets and jumpers, and keep an eye out when you're next shopping.

Get rid of anything un-mendable or too small by giving it to a friend or gifting it to charity.

Dryclean anything soiled, repair that skirt you know needs a new hemline, and replace items that are looking tired, especially around the neckline. If you don't love it or use it, it's out.

See? I bet you're feeling fresher already.

Experiment with unlikely items

Seen something worn on the street or in a shop window that takes your fancy? There will always be new trends. Many of them will not be keepers, but give things a go. Take a chance. Fluffy sheepskin slides, for example, or a daring crop top/high-waisted skirt combo, which you might feel like steering clear of with a very long stick ...

Visit shops just to browse and develop your tastes. You're busy, we're all busy, but it could be just five minutes on the way to a meeting, or an indulgent half hour spent browsing. Think of it as 'you' time.

Try on clothes and accessories before dismissing them, and you might be surprised by what you find — even if it's something you didn't think would ever work for you.

Nothing ventured, nothing gained.

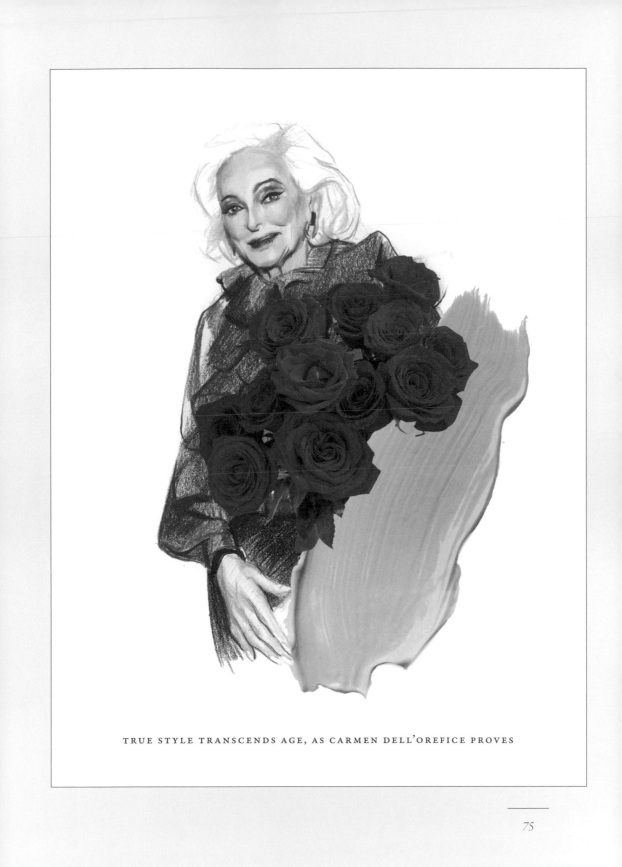

TRUE STYLE TRANSCENDS AGE, AS CARMEN DELL'OREFICE PROVES

The ins and outs of comfort dressing

There is nothing wrong with being comfortable — but try not to make it your default setting. Getting out of your comfort zone can make a huge difference to the way you feel, and the way you appear to others.

That said, don't wear things you constantly have to rearrange, pull down, feel exposed to the elements in, or are just too small for you in the first place. Nothing screams awkward like a grown woman readjusting herself, shivering in flimsy clothing or stubbornly wedging herself into a frock two sizes too small, à la Edina in *Absolutely Fabulous* (although we love her).

Examples of great high–low outfits

▶ **Creative corporate**

A beautiful designer blazer

Logo T-shirt from a sports or streetwear brand

Denim jeans

Brogues or a pair of strappy heels

▶ **Relaxed chic**

Silk print designer dress

Denim jacket (egalité!)

White leather or canvas trainers

▶ **Bohemian luxe**

Vintage or ethnic skirt from your travels

A silk blouse

Slides or wedges — nude tones will elongate your legs

Every piece tells a story

▲

Some women specifically choose their clothes because they
tell a story about who they are and where they've come from.
Sarah Jane Adams, 64, is one of them.

Born in post-war England, Sarah Jane is an antique jewellery
dealer and designer who became a model and Instagram
sensation in her early sixties.

Featured on Ari Seth Cohen's Advanced Style blog, and with
hundreds of thousands of followers on Instagram, Sarah Jane
knows exactly who she is and what she likes. As well as what
doesn't work for her. Walking past a department store's cosmetics
counter a few years ago, a sales assistant offered her a product she
promised would get rid of her wrinkles overnight. 'No thanks,' she
replied, beating a hasty retreat. 'Because I love my wrinkles. They're
my stripes, my badge of honour; a mark of who I am and where
I've been ... I wouldn't want to get rid of them.' And that's how the
hashtag #mywrinklesaremystripes was born.

Posing in a red and white Adidas jacket in a picture her husband
took, Sarah Jane's image went viral (captioned by her daughter:
'My mum looks cooler than me'). Seth Cohen saw it and got in
touch to see if Adams would be interested in meeting in person,

Ageless
Style

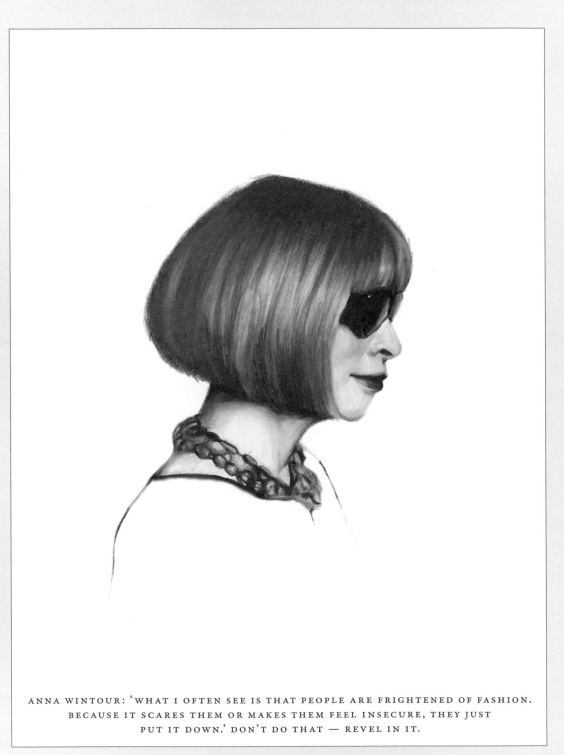

ANNA WINTOUR: 'WHAT I OFTEN SEE IS THAT PEOPLE ARE FRIGHTENED OF FASHION.
BECAUSE IT SCARES THEM OR MAKES THEM FEEL INSECURE, THEY JUST
PUT IT DOWN.' DON'T DO THAT — REVEL IN IT.

and the two became fast friends, with Cohen featuring her in his second book, *Older and Wiser*.

Sarah Jane has since become a style icon for women everywhere who appreciate individual, rebellious fashion, and her career as an international model continues to soar. She recently shot a new campaign in London with H&M, and was seen on the catwalk for Camilla at Melbourne Fashion Week.

Sarah Jane is just inimitable. With a keen interest in talking about everything that's going on in the world, her attitude to fashion — and life in general — is inspiring. That word is bandied around a lot these days, but it's true. From her punky attitude to her long, wavy grey locks and interest in staying focused through yoga, to the way she lives her life, constantly hopping between continents to spend time with her twin daughters, whom she raised on her own before meeting her partner, David, Sarah Jane has more vitality than most women half her age.

When we last met, Sarah Jane had returned to Sydney from her beloved India, and was settling back into her newly restored home (with not a shiny new item in sight). Just like her outfits, Sarah Jane's inner-city terrace is a perfect encapsulation of her eclectic personality. David stayed behind in England to renovate another of their houses, and the pair still live separately after twenty years together. 'It works for us,' Sarah Jane says, showing no sign of jetlag. Many would agree: she's living the dream.

Traditionally pairing ethnic dresses or skirts with military-inspired clothing and streetwear — particularly her beloved collection of Adidas high-tops — Sarah Jane's look is all her own. It also reflects her storied background and interests.

'People think if you dress like this you stand out, but lots of people instantly dismiss me, especially if I'm walking through the city. And that's fine. I like being invisible. One of the reasons I wear this old, tatty thing,' she says, thumbing the silk 1940s-era jacket she's had since her twenties, 'is because, as a jeweller,

'I love my wrinkles. They're my stripes, my badge of honour; a mark of who I am and where I've been ...'

▲

I'm often wandering about with thousands of dollars' worth of diamonds and precious jewellery in my pockets. Nobody would guess.' She pulls out a snap-lock bag of exquisite brooches and rings and holds them up to the light to prove her point. 'That's why I always wear clothing with loads of pockets.'

Sarah Jane has been asked many times over, why the passion for Adidas in particular?

'One of the reasons I started wearing Adidas was because, at a certain point, you start to look like a sad old hippie or a bag lady when you dress in a crazy mix of clothes. It was all about Jeremy Scott for me. When he started collaborating with Adidas, that's what I was attracted to. Many of his pieces are collector's items now. I don't wear them to look younger, but to add a different dimension and relevance to my outfits instead. It makes everything else I wear look less worn out and tatty.'

But it is her distinctive pairing of military, vintage and ethnic clothing that sets apart Sarah Jane's style.

'My father was in the military, and I was a boarding-school child in full uniform for twelve years of my life, so I often reference that, but it's more about turning the idea of a uniform on its head. It's also about comfort. Even when I was younger, I didn't shop at high-street stores or dress to look attractive. It was the days of the hippies, and everyone was wearing second-hand. If you wanted something different, it had to be old. And I didn't have the money, anyway. My style icons were always Jimi Hendrix and Keith Richards, and they wore vintage. But I grew up learning about quality and good fabrics. I'm a purist like that — things have to be either using interesting or good fabrics, or be well made.'

As an antiques dealer, Sarah Jane spent an inordinate amount of time in markets, auction houses and second-hand stores, where she would buy 'these exotic, fabulous, weird and wonderful pieces. I remember a time I bought a pair of fabric, heavily embroidered boots: it turned out they were Tibetan, and I wore them and patched them until eventually they fell apart. I still have the ties I used to wind around my shins to keep them together.'

A free spirit who loves to travel, the countries Sarah Jane has visited have also informed her look. 'When I explore I want to be respectful of the cultures I'm experiencing. I travel across borders with great ease, because I'm often invisible, blend in, or covered. People love that I'm respectful, and in turn they're respectful to me and therefore it is easy for me to engage and share amazing experiences.'

Sarah Jane's look has evolved over the years, but it's certainly one that has captured the collective imagination. 'I never wanted to be "on trend", but because I identified very strongly with these various movements and still do, I'll keep components of one vibe and bring it into the next — from one underground movement to another.'

Some time ago, Sarah Jane shot a campaign for a well-known luxury fashion house. 'I can remember being in the room and seeing all the stuff laid out ... it was covered in horrible cheap diamantés and I remember thinking, *I wouldn't pay two dollars for this stuff, let alone hundreds.*'

When so-called luxury fashion has become mass-market, the unique or one-off is so much more desirable. Which is what is implied by the idea of not always 'buying up'. Expensive doesn't always mean better. Designers make mistakes, too. We could all do well to remember that and take a leaf out of Sarah Jane's book.

Ageless
Style

Be the best-dressed in the boardroom

INTERVIEW WITH DIJANNA MULHEARN,
AUTHOR AND CO-FOUNDER OF FASHION LABEL SESTRE

▲

Being bold in the way you dress is not for everyone. Some people need to fit in. What if you're working in a conservative industry, say, or you simply like a no-nonsense look because that's your personality? Take some tips from Dijanna Mulhearn.

With decades of experience in the luxury brand sector, on brands including Prada, Ralph Lauren and the Louis Vuitton group, Dijanna continues to consult to the world's leading luxury brands to this day. The author of *Wardrobe 101* and *Wardrobe 101 for Mums,* Dijanna started her own fashion label with best friend and business partner, the curve model Ljubenka Milunovic. Sestre (Slavic for 'sisters') creates plus-size clothes with a very specific client in mind.

'We focus on women working in the corporate world,' explains Dijanna. 'Our motto is: Be the best-dressed in the boardroom.' The label Sestre was born out of Dijanna's frustration at not being able to suggest a great label for plus-size women to wear when they attended her talks or read her books. 'There was very little out there that was appropriate for businesswomen.'

As someone who understands the power of clothes and what they say about our psychology, Dijanna thinks the uniform of black that

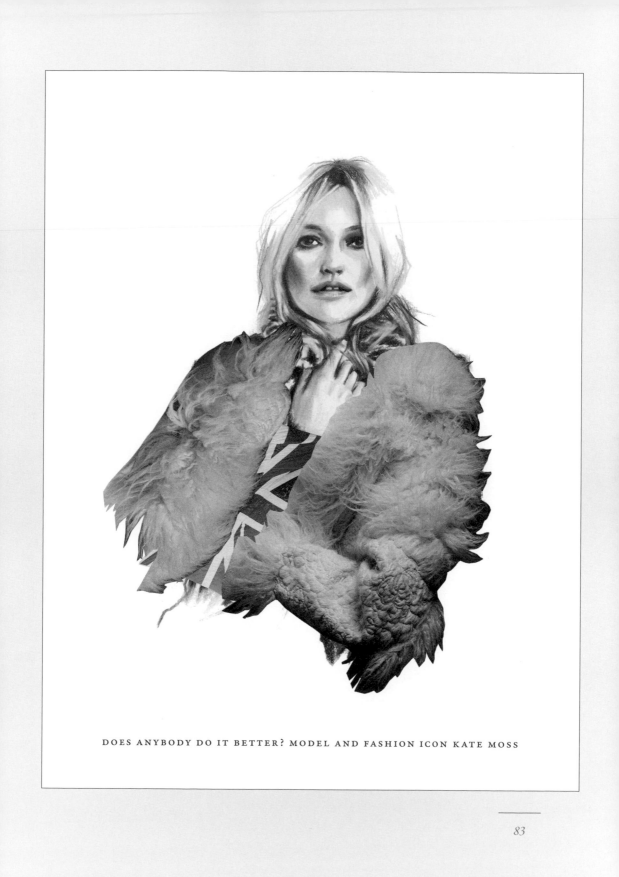

DOES ANYBODY DO IT BETTER? MODEL AND FASHION ICON KATE MOSS

some women over a certain size tend to turn to as they get older in the belief that it's slimming or flattering can be misguided.

'If you're wearing head-to-toe black, it needs to be tailored and very good quality,' Dijanna says. 'Jersey or shapeless, ill-fitting clothes send two messages out into world — you're either lazy or you're trying to hide. If you don't want to say either of those things, then you're only hurting yourself.

'Of course, it's even more critical if you're attending a job interview or discussing a promotion. You need to communicate confidence before you even secure the role. They will make a decision when you walk in the door, and be looking for ways to confirm their bias. Ask yourself, what is it you want the world to know about you? Women come in all shapes and sizes and you're blessed with the body you have, so own it. When you look your best and feel great, then you can be your true self.'

Beyond Sestre, Dijanna also creates the most beautiful, painstakingly stitched tapestries, which she attaches to the back of one-off duster coats and jackets and swaps with designer friends for their own lovingly created, unique pieces. After years of working for luxury labels, it's interesting that this designer maven has turned to more homespun crafts.

'I really believe bespoke is the new luxury. We're living in the age of the individual. In terms of status items and labels, there's no one to keep up with but yourself, and no one to impress.'

Vivienne Westwood has said that we're all buying too many clothes. Dijanna agrees. 'I have a wardrobe about this big,' she says, holding her arms a meter or so apart. 'But I have a solution for every occasion, and I wear my clothes everywhere — like this Stella McCartney jacket for example, which I'll wear to the supermarket or a meeting. I don't buy fast fashion, I only buy the best. Because it lasts forever,' she adds.

'Someone who is wearing something new every day is confused — that woman is telling the world that she doesn't know who

'I really believe bespoke is the new luxury. We're living in the age of the individual.'

▲

she is. I don't advocate shopping a lot. In my years of personal styling, I always tell women that their solutions are already hanging in their wardrobe.'

So in other words, we need to Marie Kondo the hell out of said wardrobe?

'Exactly.'

Dijanna's top 5 fashion myths, busted

Confused about what to wear and what not to wear? Dijanna shares here some of the common fashion myths worth busting.

1. **Black is universally slimming.** Black and other deep, dark colours are most effective when contrasted against something that attracts the eye. Otherwise, black is a simple silhouette that outlines every detail of your shape unless beautifully tailored. Consider a plain black T-shirt. As it's not interesting in either shape or colour, the eye searches for something interesting and goes straight to the shape underneath. Consider the same T-shirt with a colourful motif, and immediately the eye is attracted to the motif, rendering the rest of the garment insignificant. This does two things: it stops the eye on the motif rather than drawing it to the shape underneath, and it sections the T-shirt into several smaller areas rather than one wide black area. Sectioning can work in many ways to minimize the appearance of a part of your body you wish would shrink. Consider sectioning a top with a shirt and blazer combination, so that it appears as several smaller sections, or wearing a light long shirt with a high split at the sides over black pants to minimize thighs. This way, the black is invisible and other people's eyes travel exactly where you want them to.

Ageless
Style

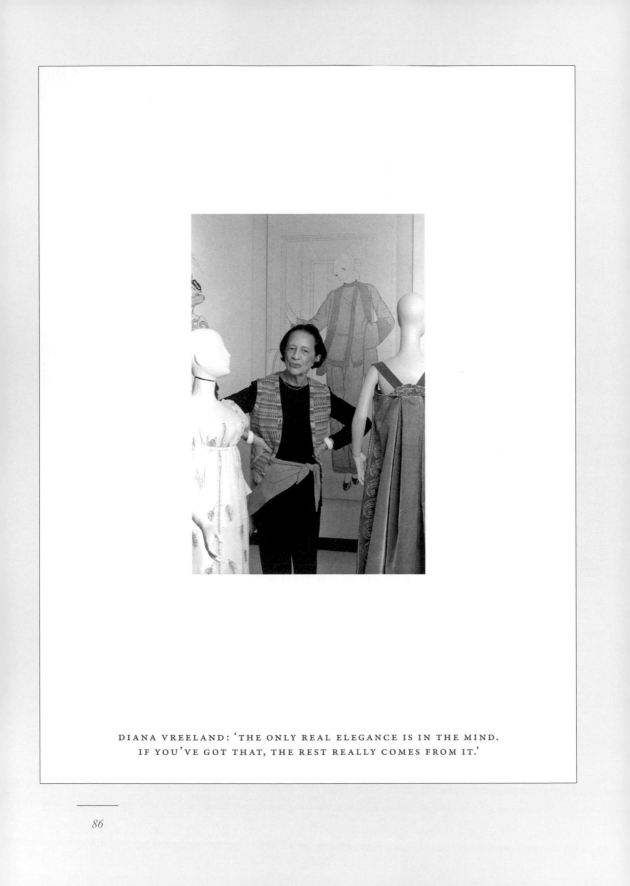

DIANA VREELAND: 'THE ONLY REAL ELEGANCE IS IN THE MIND.
IF YOU'VE GOT THAT, THE REST REALLY COMES FROM IT.'

2. **Clothes aren't important.** An increasing number of studies show that the clothing we wear affects our behaviour and performance, and certainly the way others view us or react to us. Some trivialize clothing altogether as a way of avoiding the confusion that marketing and media can create around fashion. But really, quality is key. If you look at what you spend on clothes and amortize that budget into a few select, high-quality pieces, you will be amazed at what you can afford. I always say that if you have more than four black jackets it's because you didn't buy the right one, and that goes for any garment. Look at what you keep buying, and wait for the right one, of the right quality. That way, other versions will not continue to seduce you — and though it may hurt to pay for it initially, it will save you in the long run.

3. **Body shape rules are key.** Forget the fruit! Style is not about size, and all shapes are beautiful. Iconic women in history from Diana Vreeland to Jennifer Lopez or Beyoncé have turned their unique physicality into their trademark, and you should do the same. Don't buy into body shape rules to try to reshape your body to comply with a commercial ideal. Plus, who says you should reduce the appearance of your gorgeous curves, if you have them? Wear them with pride as part of your unique shape. In addressing tricky areas of the body, there are only two things you need to consider — what is the part of your body you like the most, and what do you wish you could change? Simply highlight your favourite part with an interesting colour, shape or shine, and render your least favourite part insignificant by keeping it plain and dark. It might be as easy as big earrings or bright lipstick to draw the eye to your face, or a sporty strip down the side of your pants to highlight fabulous legs.

Contrasting colour against something quiet and creating one focal point draws the eye to the exciting part, so that it skips over your least favourite part completely. It's as simple as that.

4. **Status equals style.** Wearing a big, fancy label doesn't make you the most stylish person in the room. Using specific pieces to enhance your own unique look spells style, not dressing head to toe in a look that is dictated to you. Don't be a fashion victim. Strictly invest in high-quality pieces that work with your character; don't just buy something because it has a label — or worse, just because it's on sale. It does nothing to add to your story other than to say you spend money to impress.

5. **Only certain colours suit you.** There is in fact an orange, yellow or blue to suit everyone. It's not about whether you are 'autumn' or 'spring-toned', the secret to colour is *shade*. If you look at the items in your wardrobe that you love and feel good in, you will find that the common denominator is shade. Whether it's brights, pale, jewel-toned or muted, your shade choice is a reflection of you. If you know your shade and buy within that shade story, everything you own will go with everything else, regardless of colour. Yellow and purple are difficult to work with; however think lemon with lavender, or citrine with amethyst, and you get the picture. So, when you think of something in your wardrobe you love and never wear, it's often the shade that doesn't work with anything else in your wardrobe. If this is the case, work it back with anything else in a colour that is the same shade, or go with black and white as a fallback. Of course, there will be times when you want to break out in something different. Do that in a dress so you don't need a slew of new separates to work with.

Highlight the good

Q&A WITH LEONA EDMISTON, FASHION DESIGNER

▲

Leona Edmiston is famous for nailing dress style
for women of all shapes and sizes. First co-designer at
Morrissey Edmiston and now owner of her own label,
which she has run successfully since 2001, she has numerous
stores and followers in women of all ages.

What is it that makes a dress perfect and flattering as a wardrobe staple?
A dress is the perfect vehicle for 'highlighting the good and hiding the bad', it's the one-item outfit that simplifies decision-making, and it is the ultimate confidence-booster when you find the perfect one.

What do you think is timeless?
Fashion and trends date, but quality and style are always timeless.

What advice can you give women who might feel overwhelmed by choice or fashion in general?
It's a process of elimination to find the shapes that suit you most and the colours that make your skin glow. Once you've narrowed it down, there's no point even looking at anything else. You're just losing time, money and valuable wardrobe space.

Ageless
Style

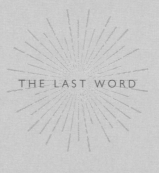

THE LAST WORD

LIVE LIFE WITH FLAIR

▲

- **Don't hide,** and don't be afraid to stand out.
- **Smile!** Keep your teeth in good shape. When you have a gorgeous smile, you light up a room.
- **Get out of your hair rut.** Consider updating your style every so often. Ask your hairdresser about colours and cuts to suit your face and complexion, especially if you're covering white or grey hair. Or consider going *au naturel* ... ask yourself, will it work for you?
- **Change up your skin routine.** If your skin or fine lines make you unhappy, there's no harm looking into good-quality serums and non-invasive laser treatments for skin rejuvenation. You're not a 'bad feminist' if you use a little Botox, just don't go overboard. Nobody wants to look like Granny Freeze.
- **Consider a makeover** if you've been doing your makeup the same way for years. Cosmetic trends and techniques change, and it's amazing how fresh you can look and feel with a few new additions. You can often book in a free session at your favourite cosmetics store.
- **Own it!** Whatever your size, height or body shape, be proud of who you are and everything you've done in life to make you, wonderfully, you. Love your body in all its glory, and others will too.

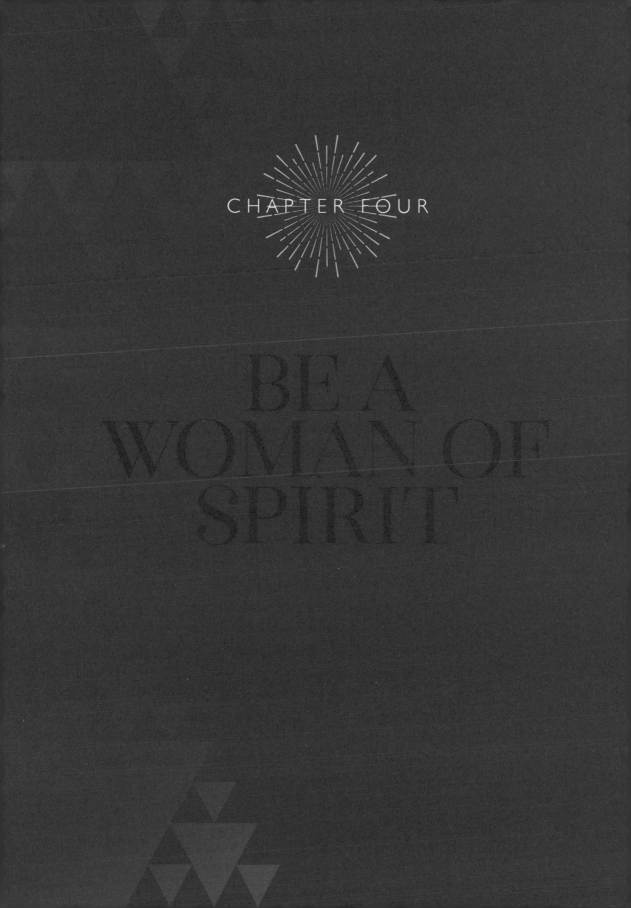

CHAPTER FOUR

BE A WOMAN OF SPIRIT

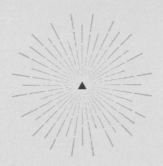

As we grow older, many of us start to wonder what the point of this whole life business is. We question why we are here and what we're meant to be doing — for ourselves as well as for others. Because at some point we do realise that it's not all about us. Deep down, we feel it: we are part of something greater.

Even if we do grow up with faith or in a religious community, spiritual depth in our fifties, sixties and seventies has a greater tenor to it — a result of living, learning and loss.

This feeling of expansiveness can come hot on the heels of a health crisis or the death of a loved one, or when children leave home and we start to reassess our role in life. As a time to reflect upon what really matters, we may wonder how we fit in the grand scheme of things. A reassessment of our inherited views on religion and spirituality can be par for the course. Have we blindly followed the faith of our parents, for example, or have our experiences shaped us to believe and behave differently? This journey informs how we face our mortality, the future and life in general.

Spirituality is one of those terms that can put people off or be considered gauche in polite conversation, but it can simply mean a faith in the connectedness of all living things, or something more refined and specific, like a religion.

Your own sense of universal laws, morality, 'good' or 'right' (although I would argue these absolute terms can be problematic) or whatever you want to call your belief system is entirely up to you. And in the spirit of coming home to ourselves — as all women of a certain age eventually do — it is yours to hold close or share with those around you as you see fit.

In this chapter, we'll hear from several remarkable women who graciously share with us their own spiritual journeys and perspectives, and explore other time-honoured practices to develop intuition and inner wisdom.

Always remain open to new ways of thinking — to be fixed is to stagnate, and to learn is to grow.

Be a Woman
of Spirit

Returning to the fold

INTERVIEW WITH JACINTA TYNAN,

NEWSREADER, COLUMNIST AND AUTHOR

▲

Sometimes, when we least expect it, life has a way of turning
full circle. Like many of us, Jacinta Tynan, 49, has spent much of her
life figuring out what spirituality means to her.

'I was raised Catholic, but always had my doubts about it. My
young and enquiring mind particularly rejected the idea that
you are born a sinner but can make amends,' Jacinta explains.

'There is a lot of guilt in Catholicism. I remember my first
confession. We had to go up to the altar and tell the priest our
"sins" but I kept thinking, I haven't done anything wrong, I'm
just a kid! I ended up making something up just so I had
something to say. So I lied in my first confession! I think some
part of me thought, there's no turning back now.

'As soon as I was old enough to have the courage to speak up —
around sixteen, I think — I refused to go to mass, which didn't go
down well with my parents. I'm one of six kids, and we all went to
mass every Sunday without fail — it was just a given. At first
I would wait until everyone sat down for mass and I would get up
from the pew and slip out the back door because I knew my parents
wouldn't want to cause a scene by trying to stop me. I'd go and sit
outside under a tree and read a book. A couple of times I refused

to leave the house, and remember grabbing on to a post and my dad trying to prize me off to get in the car and go to mass. That was the form my teenage defiance took. Other kids did drugs or got drunk, but not going to mass was my most rebellious act.'

Another thing that fuelled Jacinta's teenage anti-mass stance was the priest reprimanding her family from the altar whenever they were late. Which was often. '"Oh, we'll all just wait for the Tynans, shall we? Late again!" he'd say in his thick Irish accent,' Jacinta recalls. 'Even as a child, I realised this showed a real lack of empathy or understanding for what it was like to get six kids out the door for mass by 9 am every Sunday. Of course, the whole reason there were six kids in the first place was because of the Catholic religion. I was also quite bored as I couldn't relate to what was going on. I felt disconnected and decided that my time could be better spent reading a book.'

When Jacinta was nineteen, her first love of four years, Simon, was killed suddenly after being hit by a car. His death was difficult for her to come to grips with.

'For that to happen so young … It was a huge upheaval in my life, a huge grief. Simon and I had been together for four years and he was my best friend. It made me question everything, and sparked my first foray into what you might call spirituality, even though I didn't call it that then. I was still in touch with his mother and family who were also understandably searching for answers to try to make sense of this great loss,' Jacinta recalls.

'Simon's mother introduced me to a few books and first got me thinking about the concept of a higher power and universal law. *The Road Less Travelled* by M. Scott Peck, *The Alchemist* by Paulo Coelho and Louise Hay's *You Can Heal Your Life* were some of the first books on spirituality I read in my early twenties, and I started to look into the idea that everything happens for a reason — it was the only way I could find any meaning in losing my first love. To be able to move on, I needed to know that Simon was

Be a Woman of Spirit

still present. That I was here for a reason, and that I had known him and been loved by him for a reason, and that it wasn't all just random,' explains Jacinta.

'I haven't doubted that concept since — that we're all spiritual beings and are here to learn lessons and keep evolving. I've done a lot of reading along those lines since then and been given so many life lessons to remind me of that.'

At the age of 39 years, after a long career in journalism and just before the birth of her two sons, Jacinta discovered a new-found peace, and was drawn to meditation.

'I realised I had been seeking my whole life. I had been covering it up well, but I was pretty lost and fumbling along. I'd had depression on and off and was doing a lot of blaming — of myself and other people — for my circumstances. I was stuck in a rut and wasn't living to my full potential. When I learned to meditate, it did exactly what the brochures said it would do: I became more focused, connected and present. More conscious of who I am. Meditation has enabled me to become more connected to myself. To my truth. I realised I hadn't felt that way since I was a child — truly calm and happy and optimistic. Before I had been seeking happiness externally — from people and things and circumstances — but now I understood that I had to find it internally. I do believe there's a higher source, a universal energy. We're all connected to nature and to each other, and we can find peace by going within. I don't recognize myself from the person I was before I meditated. For me it has become the key to everything.'

Jacinta practises Vedic meditation for twenty minutes twice a day, reciting a silent mantra. Interestingly, while she doesn't regard herself as religious, Jacinta has come full circle, embracing her own Catholicism, baptising her two boys as Catholics as babies, and sending them to the local Catholic school.

'I wasn't planning to send them to a Catholic school, but it was close to home and I liked the vibe,' Jacinta explains. As a result,

'A side-effect of returning to the church is that I do feel like I belong somewhere now. I hadn't expected that.'

▲

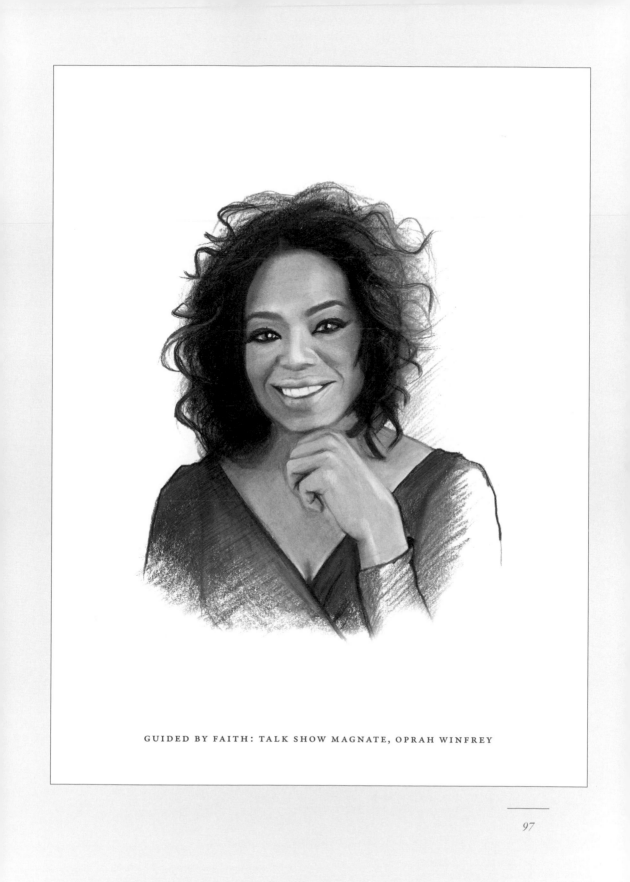

GUIDED BY FAITH: TALK SHOW MAGNATE, OPRAH WINFREY

she found herself asking some really hard questions about what this meant to her, and whether this was what she really wanted for her boys. Determined to be authentic with her intentions, Jacinta started tuning in during mass.

'I realised that everything I'd been reading in all those books for years was right there in the Bible. It wasn't a contradiction after all, but was in alignment,' Jacinta recalls.

'It dawned on me that it was possible to look beyond the religion — and some of the outdated constraints and constrictions which I don't agree with. It all made sense to me now.

'I reckon Jesus is a fine role model for my sons. Much to my surprise I find myself saying to them, *What would Jesus do in this situation?* It makes me smile to myself, as I never would have imagined it,' Jacinta muses.

When she chose to bring her boys up in the Catholic faith, Jacinta felt it would provide a good spiritual and religious basis from which to make their own decisions later.

'I make sure they're aware that this is just one religion of many, answering their questions as we go along. I let them know that Jesus is not the be-all and end-all. That he's just one of many prophets, and this is one of many religions, and they can choose what to believe as they grow up,' she explains.

Jacinta is pleased that she has actively chosen Catholicism for her kids, instead of just going along with it because she was born into it. 'I'm turning up to mass by choice and I like what I'm hearing. Jesus was a wise prophet and his teachings are still extremely relevant today — and completely congruent with many of the spiritual teachers I follow. I think I blamed him for the patriarchal system the church was when I was growing up, but I can see now that's not what he stood for.

'The church itself is still quite outdated and I don't support a lot of their views in regards to gay marriage, contraception, abortion, female priests, or the way it has historically handled

'It's all about taking the good and discarding what doesn't work for you.'

▲

sexual abuse by priests — but in terms of the content of the teachings and the sense of community, I do value it,' she says.

Jacinta particularly values the church's emphasis on forgiveness and taking responsibility for your actions.

'These are wonderful concepts for children to get so young. I don't want my kids growing up believing that they're inherently bad. But I do value the self-analysis, and that this process encourages you to take ownership of your role in things. The kids are taught to forgive and make amends — it's an invaluable life lesson,' she explains.

'Something else I have taken from the religion is the sense of social justice and giving back to the community, looking out for those who are less fortunate. That part has stayed with me since I was a child, and I'm so glad my boys are understanding the importance of that, too. It's all about taking the good and discarding what doesn't work for you.'

Don't feel the need to justify your faith.
It is yours and yours alone.

Spiritual depth has enriched me

Q&A WITH RONNI KAHN,
SOCIAL ENTREPRENEUR AND FOUNDER OF
THE FOOD-RESCUE CHARITY, OZHARVEST

▲

Born in South Africa, Ronni Kahn, 67, moved to Israel where she
lived on a kibbutz for many years, before emigrating to Australia
in 1998 and starting an events management business. While
working in corporate hospitality, she was shocked by the
amount of food waste, so she founded OzHarvest in 2004,
a non-denominational charity that rescues excess food
that would otherwise be discarded. The food is
redistributed to charities that support the vulnerable.

Are you a spiritual person?
Yes — spiritual rather than religious. For me, 'religious' means you
adhere to a particular faith, whereas 'spiritual' means it's not about
worshipping one particular god; it's a belief system that doesn't
depend on a religious system. I was brought up in the Jewish faith,
and while Judaism has a huge amount of spirituality, that's not the
side that was tapped into, in my personal experience.

Can you explain how you practise spirituality?
I have a teacher, Amma Narayani, who has helped guide my life
for the past fifteen years. He happens to be Hindu, but espouses

the philosophy that we are all one, we are all the same, and we are on this earth in order to serve, do good and make a difference.

How did you meet?

That was very interesting. My younger son, Edo, was introduced to his ideas fifteen years ago and said he was going over to India to meet him. I thought, 'Oh my god, my son's joining a cult!' I needed to check out what he was getting into, so I arrived at this ashram and was fundamentally and profoundly struck by the depth and power of a simple message: that we are here to serve, do good, and shift and change the world into the best possible place it can be.

Is this what drives your work?

I'd already started OzHarvest by the time I met my spiritual teacher, but there's absolutely no doubt the most important elements infusing OzHarvest are spirit, energy, generosity, joy, love and humanity. All of those things are informed by the fact that I do have faith.

Does the idea of God come into your spiritual beliefs?

The divine does. When we think of God, we probably think of either a white-haired person, or Jesus, or a particular embodiment of God. But the divine is in each and every one of us. That's the difference — it's about finding that.

Do you think it's important to have spiritual depth — especially as we grow older and more experienced — and why?

Speaking only for myself, I find living in the wonder of all that surrounds us gives me greater appreciation and deeper belief in the spirit and the extraordinariness of it all. I think that makes me aspire to be more compassionate, more grateful and therefore more aware of my impact on people and the planet. Spiritual depth has enriched me. Hopefully others get to experience that, or a version of that, for themselves.

'Living in the wonder of all that surrounds us gives me greater appreciation and deeper belief in the spirit and the extraordinariness of it all.'

▲

Be a Woman
of Spirit

———

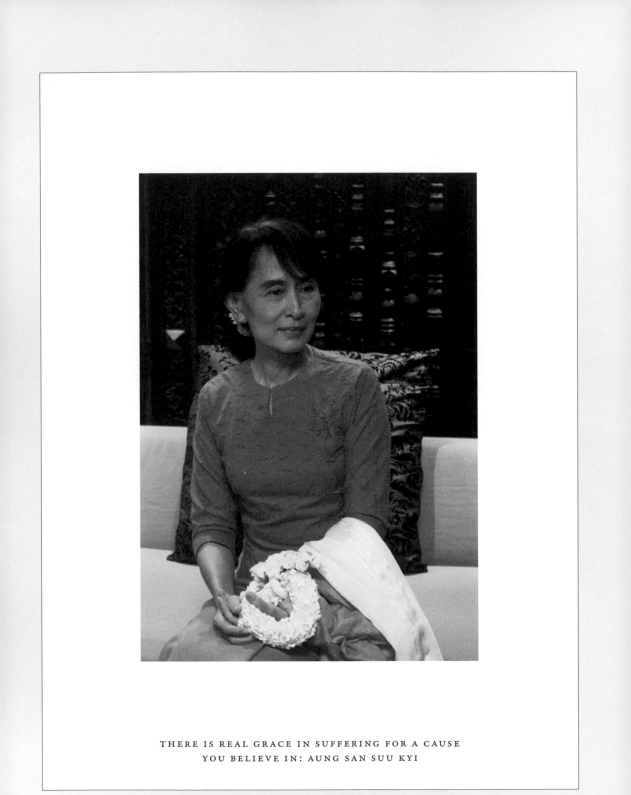

THERE IS REAL GRACE IN SUFFERING FOR A CAUSE
YOU BELIEVE IN: AUNG SAN SUU KYI

Let life unfold you

▲

For some of us, becoming a woman of spirit involves listening to and trusting our inner guidance system to set us on the right path, and celebrating the depth gained from experience. One such woman is Maggie Hamilton, 66, author of the book on sacred wisdom, *A Soft Place to Land*.

'When we're a woman of spirit, everything aligns,' Maggie explains. 'When we're connected, we have or find the tools, situations or people to help us through. Not that we don't have challenges — there's always plenty of those.'

Most of us would agree we're living in uncertain times — from the unsettling political climate to the breakdown of traditional workplaces, to our unstable economy and general family dislocation. But faith is one of those tools we can use to navigate our way through the world with more ease and grace, and it's possible to tap into it through such simple means as experiencing a walk in a park.

'I couldn't live without meditation or nature,' Maggie says. 'Daily they help connect me to all that is. Nature is a great teacher, and a book of life once you learn to read it. Silence is also essential. It's the perfect tool to get out of your head and into the wisdom of your heart.'

Be a Woman
of Spirit

For Maggie, sacred journeys are also deeply enriching. 'When we set off on a journey with holy intent, life's holiness reveals itself, allowing us to become more whole.'

Maggie says sacred journeys are about reconnecting to all that is, which in turn reconnects us with ourselves. So where are life's sacred places? 'Wilderness is nearly always sacred, because it's not muddied by our human footprint, by all the emotional and other baggage we tend to carry around,' she explains.

'I've been lucky to spend time in some of the world's great forests and deserts, in a wide range of holy places across the planet. Locations that have helped me on my journey towards wholeness, and to gift these insights to others.

'The wonderful thing is that we don't need to leave our towns and cities to experience life's sacred places. We each have locations close by that uplift our spirit. A pocket park. A small beach. A waterfall, stream or river.'

When we make a point of visiting these special places every so often with loving intent, explains Maggie, we build a bridge to all the healing available there. And, through our positive thoughts we help 'grow' the healing power of that place for others.

We don't have to spend hours in such locations, Maggie adds. 'Half an hour of quiet may be all that's needed. Then we're able to return to our routine a little more balanced, more able to treat ourselves and others well — which, I believe, is the true definition of empowerment.'

Maggie says she trusts the universe implicitly. 'Never once has it let me down. It has prompted me to make some left-of-field choices in my career and relationships, from where I choose to live to how I spend my time. Often, it's required a lot of trust while feeling wobbly (frequently the two go hand-in-hand), but the universe never nudges us to make changes to set us up — only to set us free.

'Life is more miraculous and more intricate than we can conceive. It's important to be able to spot this, even in the least lovely places and situations we find ourselves in. The quieter you are, the more profound your connection will be with all the good waiting for you there,' Maggie believes.

'Don't wait for others to approve. Let go of the need to prove. Choose instead to let life unfold you.'

Maggie's suggested spiritual reading list
Autobiography of a Yogi by Paramahansa Yogananda
The Razor's Edge by W. Somerset Maugham
The Mist-Filled Path by Frank MacEowen
Goddesses in Everywoman by Jean Shinoda Bolen
The Field by Lynne McTaggart
Romancing the Ordinary by Sarah Ban Breathnach
Women Who Run with the Wolves by Clarissa Pinkola Estés
Anam Cara by John O'Donohue
… and everything by Alberto Villoldo

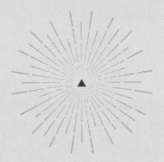

Connecting with spirit

Now that you are in your own power age, with years of rich and fulfilling life experiences under your belt, this is a wonderful time to consider and reconnect with your own spirituality. Do you still hold the same belief system you once did, or has time and experience changed it beyond recognition? What have you dispensed with along the way, and why? What does spirituality look like to you now, and what do you want it to be?

Beyond religion, here are a few of the more popular spiritual practices that may help inject a little magic and circumspection into your everyday life.

Gratitude This is the juice — the *numero uno* key to happiness. Seeing the small blessings in the things we have, and realising how truly rich our life is, definitely has the capacity to make us feel better, or whole.

If you're reading this book, I bet you're wealthy in a way that has nothing to do with your bank balance. Do you enjoy good health?

If not, do you appreciate the myriad ways your body works without you having to do anything about it, and what a miracle that is? Do you experience moments of pleasure or exhilaration when you feel relief from pain or can do something as simple as take a bracing walk? And if you're fit and able to do so much more, how much better does that make you feel?

How about the wealth of people in your life? Are you grateful for your children, grandchildren, partner, family and friends? I bet you're special to a great many of them. If you're not outgoing, how about just one or two exceptional people who accept you for who you are, and in whose company you feel cherished and safe?

What about education and experience? Two powerful tools to have in our arsenal for anything life can (and will) throw at us.

Even regrets can be useful to help us grow and perform better the next time around.

Try listing all the things you're grateful for when you fall asleep at night. It's loads better than counting sheep. Because practising gratitude raises the bar. It will also draw more people into your life, which of course gives you more to be grateful for. See? It's an awesome, self-perpetuating cycle.

Yoga I've touched on this already for its stress relief and health-related benefits, but yoga can also provide wonderful access to tapping into your latent spiritual power. Yoga was originally created by practitioners to help them go inwards and meditate better. That's why they developed the poses in the first place, thousands of years ago — to focus the mind on breath and movement, so they could drop into a deeper, more intense form of meditation.

Say *Ommmmm*.

Meditation There's no better time than now to start practising meditation. Becoming aware of the 'monkey chatter' in your mind and learning to still it is a skill worth more than gold. It's the open secret that will supercharge your Zen, and have you approaching most things in life with an enviable air of calm. Furthermore, a regular habit of meditation tends to act as a kind of 'gateway drug' to other healing modalities.

Simple discipline is the goal to aim for. Twenty minutes per day will change your life — indeed, scientists say it will change your brain — providing clarity and much-needed distance from reactionary feelings and behaviours. We're all juggling countless demands on our time, but you can *make* time for meditation when it's this important.

Psychic medium and astrologer, Jessica Adams, 54, recommends clearing a corner of your bedroom to sit with a cushion and your headphones. 'Tibetan meditation chants or music and a place for incense or an aromatherapy burner can inspire you. Get the space first, then get the headspace. You get the headspace by finding peace and quiet in your day or evening. Time alone, just for you. Then find the meditation technique or recording that works for you. There are many to choose from and there will be one that feels right.'

If you're struggling to justify the time away from other commitments, carve it out from less-nourishing activities. Limit your time on social media, for example. Think about the last time you slipped down a Facebook rabbit hole, only to look up, blinking into the light a full hour or two later. It's the very antithesis of mindfulness, and yet so many of us are guilty of it.

There are thousands of courses and resources available to teach you how to meditate, but you don't need to approach your practice too rigidly. Slot in meditation during your daily commute if you can. Meditation apps like Insight Timer and Headspace are available for you to use anywhere, anytime.

When life is so busy with family, work and technology demanding our time from the moment we wake up, it feels more crucial than ever to set a peaceful template for the day ahead in that first hour of waking. But don't be too hard on yourself if you can't get to it to

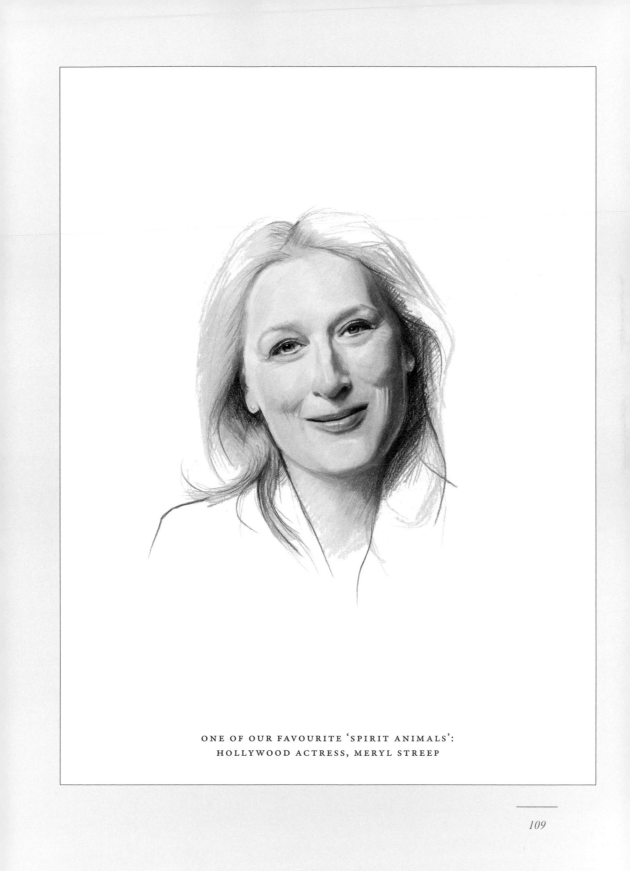

ONE OF OUR FAVOURITE 'SPIRIT ANIMALS':
HOLLYWOOD ACTRESS, MERYL STREEP

begin with. Start small and work your way up to longer meditations. Incremental steps add up, shaping our brains for the better, helping us concentrate and even solving depression. And it's free! All you need to do is close your eyes and breathe.

Speaking of breathing ... breathwork Being conscious of your breath, breathing through your nose and breathing deeply is just the trick to calm a worried mind or bring you back to a feeling of centeredness, particularly if you slow down your outward breaths.

This simple breath exercise works wonders for focusing you on the moment:

- breathe in for the count of four
- hold for a count of two
- breathe out for a count of six
- repeat.

When sleep is elusive, work your way through six rounds of these breathwork exercises. If you get to six, start again, but it's unusual that you'll make it to a third or even fourth round.

When in doubt, pause and take a minute to breathe deeply and consciously.

Manifestation

Spiritual practitioners have been following the law of attraction for years, but if you've ever given it a go, you'll know that simply wanting something desperately enough is not enough to make it instantly appear — you have to put in the legwork first.

Manifestation, explains Jordanna Levin, author of *Make It Happen*, has long been misunderstood, and has somehow been boiled down to the notion that 'thoughts become things'. But manifestation is far more than that. 'It's a by-product of respecting and listening to your inner knowing in each and every moment, and an awareness that you are the co-creator of your own future,' Jordanna explains. 'By bringing conscious awareness to your thoughts, feelings, actions and faith, you're able to manifest anything you desire.'

Jordanna says the only tool required for manifesting successfully 'is a deep belief in your own self-worth. The rest will follow. Until you can believe you're worthy and deserving of what you're trying to manifest, manifestation will escape you. This can be applied to anything you want, no matter how big or small.'

Thoughts + Feelings + Actions + Faith
= Successful Manifestation

All four parts of the above equation are integral, explains Jordanna. 'Aligning your thoughts with what you want to create, feeling what it's like to already experience that creation, taking conscious action towards making it happen, and having faith in both yourself and the support of something greater than you — that is, The Universe.'

But everything comes at a cost — that's the universal law of balance. We can manifest almost anything we want in life if we lay the groundwork, but we have to *do the work*, and manifest for our greater good and the good of those around us.

Be a Woman
of Spirit

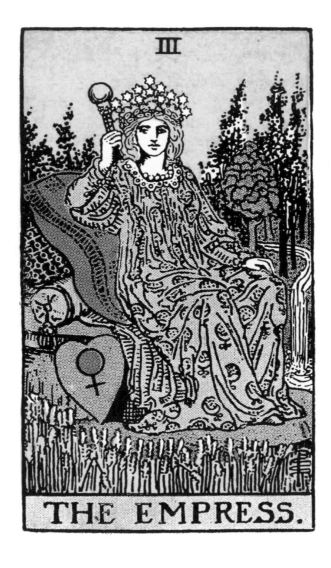

LOOK TO THE TAROT FOR INSPIRATION: THE EMPRESS
IS A CARD OF ABUNDANCE

Astrology and tarot Even if you've never been into star signs or having your tarot cards read and it all seems a bit 'out there' or counterintuitive to your belief system, there's no doubt that there has been a greatly renewed interest of late in both areas, and all things esoteric in general. Astrologer and tarot devotee Jessica Adams says that the archetypes of tarot and astrology have a lot to offer women as they enter mid- to late life.

If you have a tarot deck or can take a screenshot of tarot cards online, you can either pin these cards on a board, or use them as a desktop screensaver for inspiration:

- *The Queen of Swords* shows you the strength and force of an older woman — you don't mess with her!
- *The Queen of Coins* shows the wealth and security that comes with growing older and having property.
- *The Queen of Wands* shows a born teacher or mentor to younger people.
- *The Queen of Cups* shows a woman whose motherhood choices are behind her, who has fascinating new relationship choices.
- *The High Priestess* shows a mature woman with qualifications, certificates or degrees under her belt.
- *The Empress* shows a woman who now has the time after retirement or business success to save the planet.

And in astrology:

- *Minerva* is an asteroid relating to wisdom; the goddess who gives her name to this asteroid is always featured with an owl.
- *Diana* is the asteroid associated with the ageless goddess of the hunt, who chose not to wed or have children so she could be free.
- *Ops*, an asteroid, shows the older mother who knows how to handle every family issue.

Be a Woman
of Spirit

▶ *Ceres* is a planet in your horoscope symbolising great power in the face of change — another older mother symbol.

If you have your astrological birth chart, Jessica recommends looking for the days when the Sun passes over Minerva, Diana, Ops and Ceres in your horoscope. 'Those are the days these goddesses wake up in your chart, and using them on that day can turn your life around.'

Feed your soul
Here are some other modalities that cross over from self-care into spiritual healing.

Journaling The act of writing is cathartic and powerful. Use journaling to work out your inner thoughts, and unlock painful or knotty emotions when you're feeling 'stuck'.

Kinesiology Have you tried kinesiology? It's a hands-on treatment with a practitioner that studies the way your body responds to questions asked of you during a session. The thinking behind it is that thoughts and feelings 'lodge' in our bodies, and while we think we may have processed something that's happened to us, our body often begs to differ. Practitioners ask a question, and the body responds with an almost involuntary tic, answering yes or no. It may sound trippy to some, but others swear by it.

Acupuncture Hate needles? Acupuncture isn't the same as getting your travel shots. It's about balancing your 'chi' and fixing 'blockages' in your energy system. Sometimes intense, rarely painful, and always invigorating, acupuncture is useful for those niggling ailments which have been hanging around for too long, like neck pain or poor digestion. There's even a form of facial acupuncture which acts as a mini-facelift. True story.

The
Power Age

Womens' circles There's nothing quite so comforting as the support of a trusted group of women. The very act of coming together in a psychologically safe space is, in itself, a form of magic. Do some research on women's groups in your local area, or start one yourself with a few friends. It might surprise you how much you look forward to attending each month. Even better, time your meetings to coincide with the lunar cycle, and create a sense of ritual and symbolism around it. *Practical Magic,* anyone?

Forest bathing Look it up: it's a thing. But you don't need to make the journey into a literal forest. It simply means spending time in nature to inspire peace, gratitude and calm ... all the good feels.

Crystal healing Since ancient times, many cultures have used crystals for their powerful healing qualities. Rose Quartz for love, Amethyst for stress reduction and clarity, Black Tourmaline for protection... the list goes on. Then there's the all-rounders like clear quartz, known as the 'Master Healer'. Not only are crystals said to work energetically, but they make pretty decorative items in the form of jewellery, homewares or raw stones for display. Why not?

Sacred journeying Retreats, short workshops and trips with indigenous cultures ... you'd be amazed how many activities are available even in your local area, which can help open your eyes to the world around you and the wisdom of ancient cultures. Keep your eyes peeled — doing something outside the box once or twice a year can provide such a powerful feeling of growth and wellbeing.

Walking a labyrinth Believed to be related to wholeness, labyrinths have long been associated with meditation and journeying into the self. There's no right or wrong way to walk a labyrinth, but following a meandering and purposeful path to its center is said to unlock powerful self-healing.

FIND YOUR OWN PATH

▲

When it comes to work on ourselves, this is work that's never really done. As Clarissa Pinkola Estés writes in *Women Who Run With the Wolves*: 'When women reassert their relationship with the wildish nature, they are gifted with a permanent and internal watcher, a visionary, an oracle, an inspiratrice, an intuitive, a maker, a creator, an inventor and a listener who guide, suggest and urge vibrant life into the inner and outer world.'

But you have to do the work before the epiphanies flow thick and fast — them's the breaks. What's that saying? It won't happen overnight, but it will happen.

Wherever you sit on the spiritual spectrum, stick with it, explore, enjoy ... the journey is entirely up to you.

CHAPTER FIVE

WANDERLUST

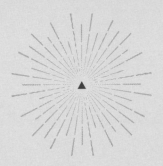

It's said variety is the spice of life, and nothing disrupts our routine or sets us dreaming as much as travel does. Some of us are lifelong globetrotters, some just dipping our toes into travel for the first time now that the kids are grown, but one thing is certain: the older we get, the more opportunity there is to travel *well*. And I don't mean at great expense, or even in great style (although that can be lovely, too) — but with a sense of what's meaningful and how we like to best spend our days.

Are you a cocktails-on-the-beach, poolside lounger type, or do you prefer exploring foreign cities on foot and mixing with the locals? Are gourmet delights your passion, or are you more of a thrill-seeker who likes to indulge in skiing, mountain-bike riding or sailing? Would no trip be complete without a visit to art galleries or a walk around ancient ruins, or do you prefer going offline and getting totally lost in nature? Do you consider yourself not properly *au fait* with a culture until you've lived there?

Preferences change as we mature, and you may have been any one — or all — of these types of travellers at different points in

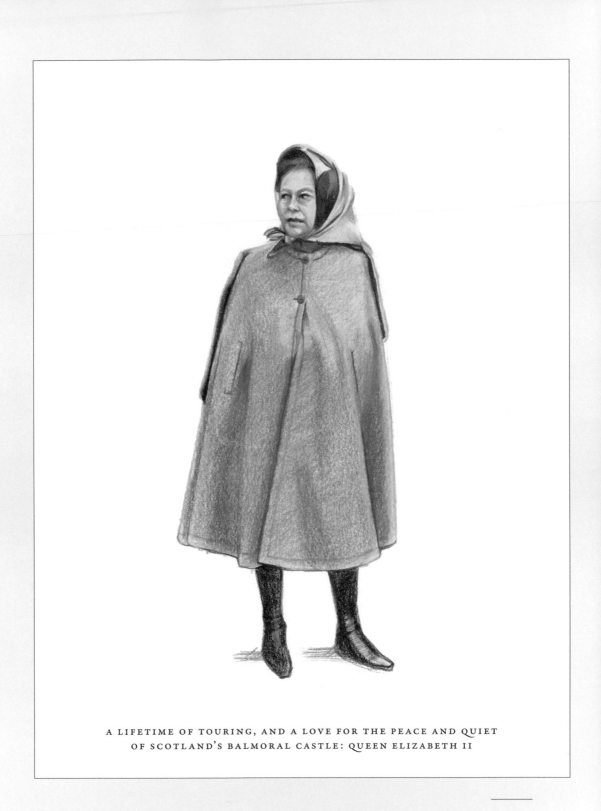

A LIFETIME OF TOURING, AND A LOVE FOR THE PEACE AND QUIET
OF SCOTLAND'S BALMORAL CASTLE: QUEEN ELIZABETH II

your life. There is no better time to celebrate the opportunities that each decade brings.

Travelling can be a pure joy. It can also be confronting, infuriating or truly life-changing. Sometimes all of the above in one amazing, jam-packed trip. Things can unravel surprisingly quickly when problems occur, but even that prompts a reassessment and an opportunity to learn, accept and evolve — after which, we're never quite the same.

Staying at luxury resorts every time you travel won't open you up to new or truly authentic experiences. Go off the beaten track to experience how other cultures live. Stay awhile. If you're lucky enough to travel overseas, you're one of the world's most fortunate people anyway, so appreciate it. Learn, explore and do things you never have before. Then come home with fresh eyes, ready to take on the world anew. This is travelling at its finest.

Travelling for good

If youth is for experimentation, then the later years in life are all about focusing on what really matters and spreading your wings in new ways.

There are so many travel possibilities. Why not choose a surprising destination, or think about ways to take a longer getaway? You could even try looking into a volunteer vacation.

After a successful career in marketing for various arts bodies, Vanessa, 72, decided that she didn't want to retire only to spend her time meeting with friends for coffee mornings or taking up golf — she wanted to make the next decade of her life really count. With no children of her own, Vanessa spent most of her working life devoted to her job, friends and her relationship, and had been minimally involved in a charity organisation helping homeless families and children in Asia.

After discussing it with her husband, Richard, she decided to take six months out to live in Cambodia and help build a village.

'I knew it was the right time,' says Vanessa. 'It was something I'd long been interested in, but it seemed so far from my experience of working and commuting and living in the city for most of my life. We'd donated money before, but I always felt that I'd like to do more, given the chance. So I looked into volunteer options for an extended period.'

Vanessa was 64 when she made her first trip. It was eye-opening. 'There were displaced families living very tough, with little access to clean water or anything you and I take for granted,' Vanessa explains.

'We built basic shelters with them, helped cultivate vegetables, and provided medicine for the children. In such a tropical climate, bacteria spreads quickly and a small cut can become dangerously infected overnight, but the people are resilient.

'I can't really explain what a privilege it is to be there — with so little of what you and I consider necessary, they had such appreciation and joy for life. It's taught me a lot about what we value and what we really need.'

In the past eight years, Vanessa says she has spent more time travelling back and forth to Asia than in England, her home country. Now, Richard comes too.

'We travel around, but tend to base ourselves somewhere for a season,' she explains. 'It's certainly not the retirement we were expecting, but it works. At some point, we probably will need to stop as our health changes, but we've been very fortunate so far. I had a bout of dengue fever about five years ago, but went home to recover and eventually returned. It will be difficult to return to England full-time. Living like this changes you.'

Making lovely memories

After working very hard on their recruitment business with her husband for many years, Sally, 67, now travels on international getaways each year. Recently she has started inviting her daughter Skye along, as well as her son-in-law and grandchildren.

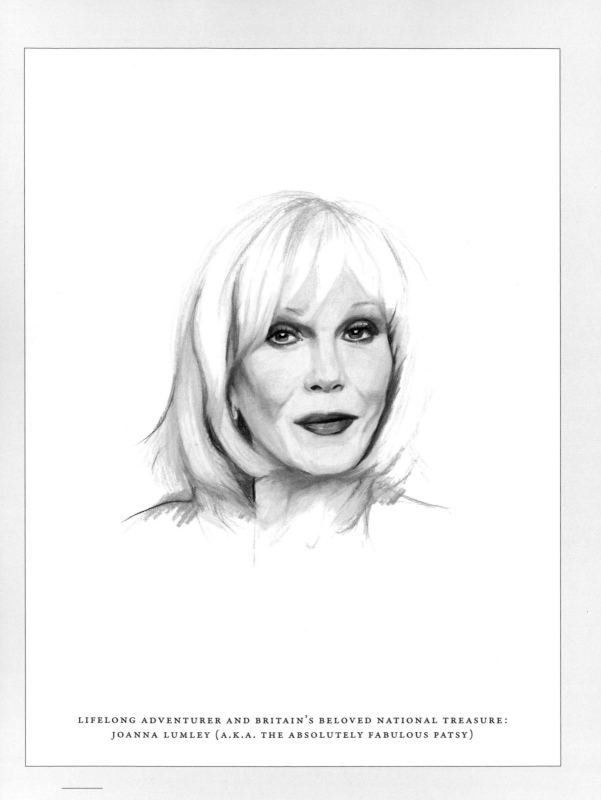

LIFELONG ADVENTURER AND BRITAIN'S BELOVED NATIONAL TREASURE:
JOANNA LUMLEY (A.K.A. THE ABSOLUTELY FABULOUS PATSY)

'When our children were young,' explains Sally, 'we didn't really have the time or the money to travel overseas. But then we sold the business a few years ago, and started travelling quite a lot. It was liberating, finally visiting all the places we'd dreamed of, without having to rush back home.'

Sally and her husband took a six-week cycling trip in Vietnam, following the Mekong River, and Sally recently travelled to southern France with her daughter to take a local cooking course.

'Skye has two small children and a full-time job — she's at that stage in her life where it's hard to get away,' says Sally. 'But I wanted to take her somewhere to celebrate her fortieth birthday. It was such a beautiful trip. We had three weeks together, just the two of us — I don't remember ever spending so much time alone together before, not since she was small.'

Travelling with her daughter had its moments, admits Sally. 'We both like to do things our way, and it's not always easy sharing a room with your grown daughter — but it was a really special time,' she recalls. 'I'm glad we were able to do it. I think we both have some lovely memories.'

Off-trail adventures

It's not always easy to choose the right travel partner. Even close friends or loved ones can be challenging to travel with, or might not have the time or capacity to do so.

Generally quite happy to travel alone, Belinda, 74, effectively 'advertises' through Facebook and her circle of friends for a travel partner when she feels like company.

'I'm divorced and I don't have children, and many of my friends aren't interested in visiting the sorts of places I like to visit,' Belinda explains.

Travelling extensively throughout the Middle East and several times to Syria, Belinda is not afraid to visit travel destinations with a security warning, although she finds that other people often are.

'After years of doing this, I've met some people like me, but they don't live in the same country as me,' Belinda explains. 'When I'm thinking of going somewhere, I put a call out on Facebook and there's usually someone I met once, or a person one of them knows, who will be in the same place at the same time.

'We meet for a day or more, but generally I travel alone. The places most people like to vacation hold no interest for me — going off the tourist trail is more adventurous, and you learn more.'

The world is your oyster

Travel doesn't always have to take place in retirement or when work no longer matters — can you arrange to work remotely, for example, or take a leave of absence? You might think the world will fall apart if you're gone for a month, but will it really? Set a savings goal, plan your trip and work towards the time away. And it's just an idea, but what about keeping a folder or bucket list of dream destinations? That way, you'll have something to work towards. It's always good to keep dreaming.

The following pages feature conversations with three impeccably stylish, trailblazing women: Gene Sherman (a South African), Lone Jacobsen (a Dane) and Sarah Jane Adams (an Englishwoman) who have travelled — and continue to travel — the world for very different reasons. While all differ in their worldviews, there are obvious correlations between their stories, first and foremost the importance of travelling to experience a place on a deeper level, rather than as a mere 'tourist'.

There's a whole world out there

▲

Travel and emigration are so often enriching, even in the face
of difficulties. Many immigrants end up creating a better life for
themselves and their children, but it's never easy, and can often feel
like your heart lives between many homes. For Gene Sherman, 72,
a lifetime of travelling has only sharpened her cultural curiosity.

'I feel I was a global citizen of the world, long before the term
was coined and in circulation,' says Gene. 'I'm restless if I'm in a
place for more than a few months.'

Born and raised in South Africa, Gene moved to Sydney,
Australia, in 1976, where she was awarded a doctorate in French
literature. With her rich multicultural upbringing and multi
lingual skills, she later became Head of Languages at the private
girls' school, Ascham.

After 17 years of teaching and research, Gene founded Sherman
Galleries, a leading art gallery in Sydney focusing on contemporary
artists from Australia, the Asia-Pacific and the Middle East.
Gene continues to exert her artistic influence with her latest
venture, the Sherman Centre for Culture and Ideas, which looks
to global fashion and architecture influencers to provide a vibrant
platform for the exchange of ideas.

Wanderlust

Married with two children and six grandchildren, Gene continues to live in Sydney, while travelling the world for much of the year.

'It all comes back to my family and the way I was brought up. I'm Jewish — originally Austrian from Vienna on my father's side, and Lithuanian under Russian rule on my mother's, but my parents were both born in South Africa,' Gene explains.

'I feel I was a global citizen of the world, long before the term was coined.'

▲

'English is my mother tongue, although many languages formed part of my daily experience; my father was a bilingual Afrikaans speaker and my grandmother and family spoke several languages. My father collected art and Persian carpets. He was an extraordinary man, raising us with the idea that the world was a much larger place. He was also of the opinion that girls can do anything and didn't necessarily need to marry or have children, which was unusual for his generation. How could I not have been curious about travelling, growing up in this family?' Gene muses.

'I was encouraged to be independent. As soon as I was old enough to travel by myself, my father said, "Off you go".'

With trouble spreading in South Africa, Gene was sent to Paris to stay with her grandmother, a creative and talented seamstress, one summer when she was only sixteen years old — an experience she credits as inspiring her interest in fashion and architecture.

During World War II, the French branch of her family underwent turbulent times. Many of them died in Auschwitz, at the hands of the Nazis. 'Fear of the other is a very real and natural part of the human psyche,' says Gene. 'There are a lot of people who hate in the world.' Having travelled extensively through countless countries and cultures during her life, xenophobia is something that still baffles Gene. 'It exists, but there's no rational basis for most fears relating to difference.'

As part of the Jewish diaspora, many members of her family looked outwards, appreciating what was going on in the wider world. 'One of my uncles in France lived in Paris, but had built a house in the Japanese ryokan style, with a pebble garden.

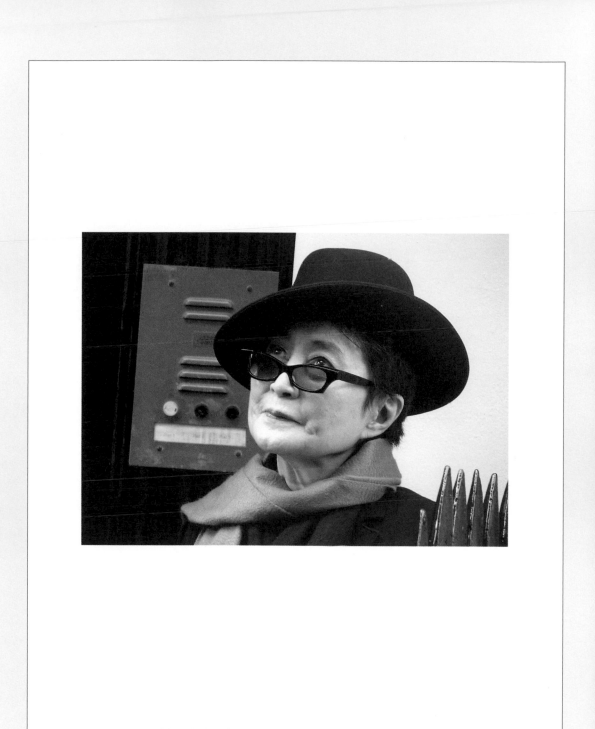

ARTIST, PEACE ACTIVIST AND GLOBE-TROTTING
SINGER-SONGWRITER, YOKO ONO

He came home for lunch each day, where my aunt would present a five or six course meal at the table in the traditional French style. After a siesta, he would head back to the atelier he worked at in the afternoon.'

In 1964, when Gene was eighteen, her family left South Africa, bound for Melbourne — a trip Gene says 'finished my family off'. After the high adventure of the journey, on a Dutch merchant ship with 'dashing and attentive naval officers', stopping in Singapore, Bangkok and Hong Kong, their final destination proved sobering.

'Apartheid was a terrible system, but Melbourne in the 1960s was deeply conservative. It felt like the end of the earth. Shops closed at 12 pm on Saturdays, whereas Johannesburg had been very sophisticated and wealthy,' Gene recalls. The family returned to South Africa only a year later, a move that 'totally humiliated' her father, given his anti-apartheid views. And tragically, feeling guilty for her failure to make a go of emigration, Gene's mother committed suicide, when Gene was only 20 years old.

'That trip was a lesson in humility,' Gene recalls.

Back in Johannesburg, Gene met and married her husband Brian, a stockbroker. As newlyweds, they planned to move to France, but after a job offer fell through they emigrated to London instead, where Gene taught French at Watford Grammar. 'I loved London — but then tragedy struck.' Her father begged her to come home, because her brother had gotten mixed up in drugs. 'My brother died of a drug overdose not long after I returned.'

Brian and Gene's two children, Ondine and Emile (the Oscar-winning producer of *The King's Speech*) were both born in South Africa, when apartheid was in full swing. With their infant children in tow, the Shermans moved to Sydney in 1976, to the artsy inner-city suburb of Paddington, which felt far more progressive and accommodating than Melbourne had just over a decade earlier.

While they were still very small, Gene left her two children in the care of her mother-in-law, and travelled to France to research her doctorate. 'The guilt at leaving them was tremendous,' she admits, 'but I felt I couldn't turn down the opportunity.'

Then, when they were much older, Gene started travelling again.

'I've been to Japan 56 times since 1987. China, Korea, Vietnam, Cambodia, Indonesia, the Philippines ... all special cultures in rapid transformation, and all favourite places to visit. I saw the shift occurring away from European culture and languages. Largely because of its proximity to Asia, and aided by its extraordinary mix of cultures, Sydney had become a major world center, which is why I opened the Sherman Galleries, with its Asian art focus,' Gene explains.

'But there is a whole world out there,' she adds. 'If you don't travel, how can you tell what's happening? I truly believe that you can't understand another culture unless you spend time in it and learn the language. For me, that's what travelling is all about. It's a very personal experience.'

A minimalist marvel: Gene's travel wardrobe

Long ago, Gene devised the perfect capsule wardrobe for her peripatetic lifestyle. Needing to simplify, she came across the 'great Japanese triumvirate': designers Issey Miyake, Comme des Garçons and Yohji Yamamoto.

'Back in 1985 when I started wearing these clothes, they were only available in black, so of course everything went together, and I found I could pack in 5 minutes. Even at home, I only have 32 hangers in my wardrobe, so everything I own fits on those. Apart from undershirts and other small, layering pieces, I only have 32 items — all from my favourite designers, all in black, and I don't wear dresses, only separates. I also splurge a bit on bags and shoes and don't wear heels, only flat shoes. It makes it easy to get dressed or throw on the perfect outfit, wherever I am.'

Wanderlust

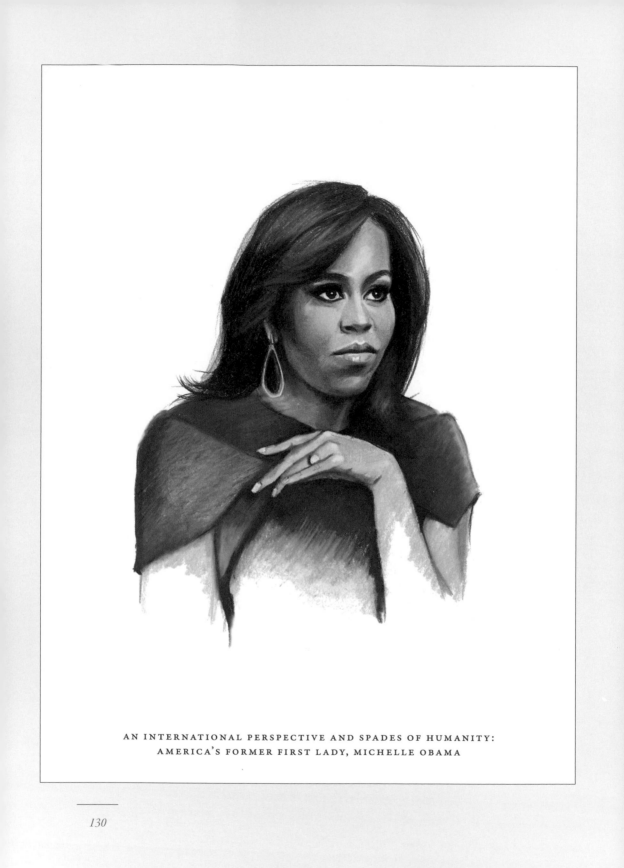

AN INTERNATIONAL PERSPECTIVE AND SPADES OF HUMANITY:
AMERICA'S FORMER FIRST LADY, MICHELLE OBAMA

Travelling is in our blood

INTERVIEW WITH LONE JACOBSEN,
DESIGNER AND RETAILER

▲

Lone Jacobsen, 50, has lived and worked all over the world for most of her life. In her late teens, she backpacked around Australia, New Zealand and the United States, meeting her husband, Søren, not long after returning to her native Denmark.

At the time, Lone was a part-time bartender studying special needs education, and Søren was working in information technology. They were polar opposites, but knew, even then, that they would always be up for adventure together.

A few years after they met, Søren was offered a job in Switzerland and lived across the border in France. Lone followed. They had their first child, a son, in Geneva, then a daughter after moving back to Denmark. After a decade of relative stability, they decided to mix it up again by moving to New Jersey, close to New York, and are now settled in Australia with their daughter, while their son is studying in Denmark. Their dream is to one day retire to Tuscany or somewhere in Spain.

'We lived in the same house outside Copenhagen for ten years while the children were small and I was working as a special needs teacher. Then a position became available in New Jersey. By that stage I was forty, and the kids were nine and twelve. I had started

Wanderlust

131

my own business with a friend — a fashion and homewares store where we also sold products we designed and made ourselves — but I couldn't give up the opportunity to move to the States.'

They never said no to Søren's work offers, and Lone says this enthusiasm for fresh experiences has shaped them.

'It made us who we are. My inner self is still the same, but it's made me a different person. I was never very good at being alone, but over the years living in different countries has given me more appreciation for my own company. It's made me smarter and more intelligent, and definitely more outgoing. And it's given our kids a life gift — the ability to adjust to different cultures and live anywhere. It really has formed them as well.'

Whenever they moved, Lone always made sure they were considering the family as a whole. 'Some children would not be good with moving so often — you have to look at their unique personalities. But we asked them lots of questions to make sure they didn't feel rootless. My son doesn't feel completely Danish, or American either, despite spending so much time there. If anything, he feels Swiss because that's where he was born.'

Lone says the age at which you move does have an impact on how easy it is to make friends or settle in.

'When we first moved to France, I was so young and it was very different to what I was used to. I found it hard. I was very lonely. In some ways, it's the hardest move I ever made. I didn't speak French, and the people I met seemed to have different personalities. Geneva was easier. We lived in a very international area with lots of Dutch, Scottish, French and Danish people — our friendship group alone covered nine different nationalities. We also met people through our Danish church.

'Moving to a new country is difficult on both a mental and physical level. It challenges you so much — but when you're in the middle of it, you're not overthinking it, just doing. When I was younger and raising my family, having stylish furniture and a home

'Living within different cultures has satisfied my curiosity for the world. It certainly makes you more open-minded and tolerant.'

▲

was everything, but I've realised that money truly doesn't buy happiness. I've had so many beautiful things in my life, but I have often had to downsize and practise non-attachment. This,' she adds, 'has made me a lighter person.'

For Lone and her family, travelling is a way of life. 'Travelling is in our family and in our blood. For me, it's very important to respect the different types of personalities in this world. It doesn't matter what your background is — if you're inspired, that's good. Living within different cultures has satisfied my curiosity for the world. It certainly makes you more open-minded and tolerant.'

Travel is expansion — it can't help but open our eyes to the world around us.

My favourite places are those that challenge me

INTERVIEW WITH SARAH JANE ADAMS, JEWELLERY
AND ANTIQUES DEALER, MODEL AND AUTHOR

▲

After a long love affair with India and a lifetime spent travelling, Sarah Jane Adams, 64, author of the memoir *Life in a Box*, says her purpose for travelling is to immerse herself in different cultures and experiences.

'There's a big difference between travel and vacationing,' explains Sarah Jane. 'For travel, my favourite places are those that challenge me.

'India used to be that for me, but now I know it so well, I spend time there for different, family reasons. Once you've been to a place and found what it is you think you're searching for, the purpose of your visits change. I continue to travel because I'm always searching for something — sometimes work-oriented, sometimes not, and sometimes I don't really know what it is.'

First visiting India in her twenties, Sarah Jane says what initially drew her there was the warm weather, the opportunity to explore and experience a completely different culture, as well as cheap living and healthy eating. 'Working in the street markets in London, I needed to escape the harsh long winter months, and the fact that it wasn't expensive to stay for extended periods meant India was a good destination,' she explains.

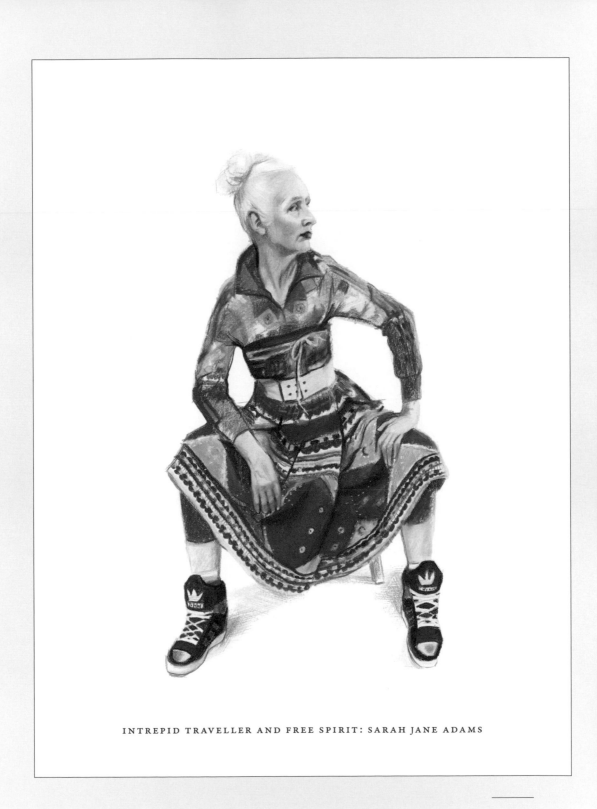

INTREPID TRAVELLER AND FREE SPIRIT: SARAH JANE ADAMS

'When I'm travelling, wherever it may be, I like being incognito — that's my comfort zone. I'm at my most comfortable when I'm blending in or being totally ignored. Blending in to the extent that you become accepted by the local people, to me is the very best thing. For me, travel strips things back so I can connect with real people and experience things at a grassroots level. I love the simplicity of that,' Sarah explains.

'I don't like to be spoiled, and I like experiencing new challenges. When I visit a different place, I can observe quietly and gently. Also respectfully. One of the good things about travelling as an older woman is that I am more easily able to connect with the local people. Oftentimes when we women are young, we don't necessarily understand fully the concept of mutual respect. We dress, or behave, in an inappropriate manner, or we think everyone wants to take advantage of us, but I'm happily at another stage of my life.'

Recently in Kashmir, Sarah Jane spent the entire time 'completely covered up', and sensed the locals appreciated it. 'I do this not only as a mark of cultural respect, but also because being invisible within another culture is a good way to learn about things. My husband, David, feels the same — we take public transport wherever we go, stay in low-key hotels and eat local, mainly street food. We explore on foot the entire day, starting early most mornings and only coming back to wherever we're staying to sleep. Yes, it can be exhausting, but I've never really had vacations. I'd be bored shitless on a vacation.'

Sarah Jane prefers to travel on a shoestring budget. 'To me, that's the most real. I'd rather have that than the luxury five-star experience. That's not travel as far as I'm concerned — it's a vacation. I occasionally take a day or so of 'vacation' within a trip. That's when I'll find a place where I can regroup, wash my clothes, repack and be ready to go again. Martinis on the beach is my idea of hell.'

When we think about vacations, it's usually in comparison to everyday life — most people feel they need an escape when they're working full-time, or are in the middle of busy child-rearing years.

'For me, travel strips things back so I can connect with real people and experience things at a grassroots level. I love the simplicity of that.'

▲

Sarah Jane says she did take her twin daughters 'on a sort of vacation to Goa when they were young, but that's not the way I travelled pre-children, or now. I feel fortunate that I've constructed a good life, so I've never really felt the need to escape it. To do something where you're *meant* to be having a good time just fills me with anxiety — I feel trapped in a bubble.'

A punk in the 1970s, Sarah Jane stays true to her anarchic roots, always choosing to take the more challenging route. 'It's part of the reason I travel the way I do. We live in different times. The world seems so bland now. I didn't do things the same as most women of my generation back then, and I don't do things the same as most women of my generation now. It's the way I stay vital.'

It's so important to learn about how other people live — it's a surefire way to spark appreciation and compassion for ourselves and others.

Travelling light with Sarah Jane

After many years of experienced travel, sometimes for months at a time, Sarah Jane has crafted a genius approach to packing.

'I lay my clothes out on the bed like a mandala, and then decide on a colour theme. What I pack depends on whether I'm going on a work trip or travelling for myself, and naturally I consider the climate and what sort of functions I'll be attending.

'Generally, I don't like to travel to cold climates (where I need winter clothes), as I prefer to travel light. People are often surprised, because I can live for months out of one suitcase. I take things that can be worn in a variety of ways — scarves are an essential, also items that can be reversed or worn in different ways.'

Sarah Jane says the first thing that always goes into her suitcase is a nail scrubbing brush, 'because cleanliness is essential', then basic underwear and comfortable, covered, stretch-cotton sleepwear. 'Regardless of where I travel, I don't ever take any medicine — apart from some herbal patches for the baker's cysts which I very occasionally get on the back of my knees (too much walking in the wrong shoes!). And I always pack earplugs and an eye mask so I can sleep wherever.

'Then I'll make a mandala colour wheel of clothes on the bed. I'll have a group of "bottoms" — trousers and skirts, which I'll colour code (say, red, orange and brown) — then I'll bring in some highlight colour touches, perhaps purples and pinks, and look for the right shades of tops to match. I'll select the scarves, dress tops and other accessories, which are all laid out in categories within a circle. I've always got two or three belts because they provide the "anchor" in my clothing, but sometimes I'll include other items which can also double as a belt. Everything can be worn, used as an accessory, and multipurposed.'

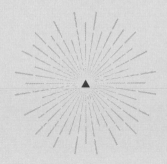

Tips for the grown-up traveller

Remember when you were young, footloose and fancy-free, with barely enough cash in your pocket to do the things you wanted, but seemingly unlimited time at your disposal? Those days are probably gone. If you're still working, time will be precious, so doing your research is especially vital.

On trips longer than a month or two, it's wonderful to follow your nose and see where life takes you. But when you only have a short amount of time away from work or family commitments, you don't want to waste it fussing about with poor accommodation, dodgy restaurants or packed tourist sites. Ask like-minded friends for their favourite places to eat and stay and visit. By this stage in life, you will have amassed a good pool of knowledge between you to share and inspire. Any conversation that starts with, 'Ooh, remember that little family bistro we went to on the outskirts of X, where they pointed us towards the old town and we somehow got caught up in a parade, and those people invited us home for tea?' is a good place to start.

Wanderlust

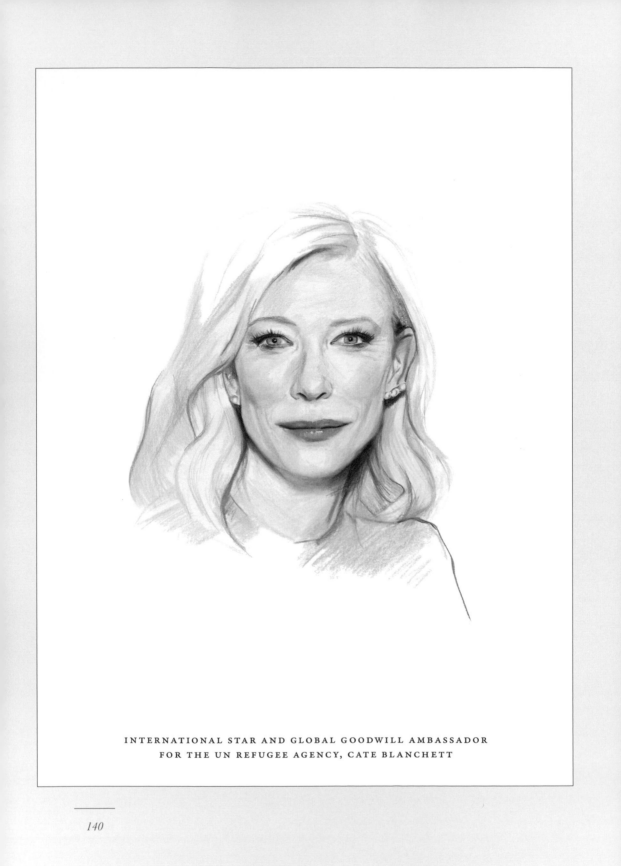

INTERNATIONAL STAR AND GLOBAL GOODWILL AMBASSADOR
FOR THE UN REFUGEE AGENCY, CATE BLANCHETT

Cross-reference your shortlist, but take with a pinch of salt some of the reviews you read on some travel sites — have you ever noticed how they always seem to feature either glowing or negative comments? 'Gorgeous! Couldn't have been better' versus 'Hated it — avoid like the plague!'? It can be overwhelming and confusing. Miserable reviewers have an axe to grind, and it's hard to trust the good ones — they might be the owners or the business or their well-meaning friends!

Don't leave home without a few good ideas about what you'd like to do at your chosen destination, so you can set off on the right foot. And check out the tips below.

Invest in travel guides Search out guides that appeal to your particular interests to help fine-tune your plans — these could be anything from 'South America on a Shoestring' by the Lonely Planet team to high-end handbooks like the Luxe or Wallpaper Guides for major cities, which include a good dash of the best shopping and culture hotspots for when you're feeling flush, or wish to take a break from hardcore sightseeing and adventure.

Enjoy the anticipation Half the pleasure in a really great trip comes from the planning and excitement as you look forward to going away. Psychologists say we actually appreciate things more in life when we anticipate them. Spontaneity is important, but relish the lead-up to your trip as part of the experience as a whole, rather than wishing the time away before you hop on that plane.

Be prepared If you find it hard to sleep when you're away, always pack an eye patch and pair of earplugs, and maybe also download a meditation or white noise app on your phone to help you get some shut-eye. Travelling isn't fun when you're too exhausted to go out and explore, although if you're the sun-lounger type, you'll probably be okay. And don't forget to pack sunscreen, bug repellent

Wanderlust

and painkillers, as finding particular medications or even an open pharmacy in a foreign place can be a nightmare. If you've ever tried buying specialist lady products from a Marrakechi pharmacist through a complex game of charades and using schoolgirl French, you'll know what I mean.

Don't overpack It's arduous traipsing to and from airports and hotels with too much luggage, especially on longer trips. Make it easy on yourself by packing sparingly, packing carefully — and if you think you can go without it, leave it at home. A good trick is to pack a week or two beforehand, then slowly whittle down your belongings as you get closer to your departure date, so you can be one badass nomad when it comes time to skip town. Besides, if worse comes to worst, you can shop for a little something to bring home as a special reminder of your trip.

Take a small touchstone If you're an unsettled traveller, take a touchstone or comfort item. Maybe it's as simple as a photograph, a scented travel candle, or a journal and pen. It could be your favourite novel, or even an actual crystal or stone. The point is to pack something familiar or comforting when everything else around you seems strange and, well, foreign. Especially good if you're travelling alone.

Sort out your visa, travel insurance and life admin Check in advance if you need any special visas for the countries you are planning to visit, and keep an eye on any travel security alerts for those areas that might negate your travel insurance or change your plans. Many vacations have been ruined by lost luggage, cancelled flights and last-minute health emergencies. Don't add to your financial burden as well — do the smart thing and find appropriate insurance cover before you leave. It's worth the extra cost for the peace of mind.

If you're planning to be away from home for a long period, let at least one person know your travel itinerary and emergency contacts for ageing parents or children, and make sure your bills will be either auto paid or emailed to you. Arrange to have all mail and newspapers collected by a neighbour or friend until you return.

Go with the flow When you finally do arrive at your destination, trust your gut and let it take you where it will.

There's simply no point stressing when flights run late or there are delays. When accommodation doesn't meet your expectations or the weather refuses to play along, there's often a silver lining, if you can only change your perspective. Embrace the unknown, appreciate the unexpected and stay chilled. Close your eyes and breathe deeply. Some things will always go pear-shaped, but you're going to enjoy yourself far more if you roll with the punches in life.

Embrace the unknown, appreciate the unexpected and stay chill.

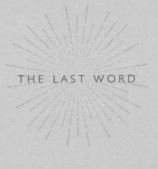

FOR THE LOVE OF TRAVEL

▲

▸ **Seize the moment and make memories to last.** Try that special the waiter is banging on about, take the scenic route, strike up conversations with strangers (remember: friends you haven't met yet!) and buy the dress. You know, the one you've fallen in love with in the window of that little boutique on the cobblestoned square? Pack your trip with varied memories that will make you smile, laugh and blush well into your twilight years, even if you're already in your twilight years.

▸ **Remember to let yourself dream.** Look in the windows of real estate agents, talk to the locals and get a proper feel for your favourite places every time you visit. Would you come back here again? Could you see yourself living here for an extended period? Would you even, given the chance, pack up and move your life?

▸ **Open yourself up to the possibilities of experiencing the world totally differently.** After all, you only live once.

CHAPTER SIX

CONNECTION & SEX

No one is an island; we are all social creatures at heart. Even when we're single, we women thrive through our relationships with others. Friendship, family and *amours* give life a richness and depth that is impossible to achieve solo. Think of all the great works of literature, music, cinema and art: they are all about relationships, at their core.

Connection is what drives us and makes us human; the stuff of life. And if love is the true basis of everything we value, our connections provide us with a solid foundation to build a meaningful existence upon.

Women know how to love. We're used to giving so much of ourselves, both emotionally and physically — sometimes to the point where we may feel there's little left. It's why we may be more susceptible than men to anxiety and certain illnesses, but also why we often remain at the center of most households, workplaces or friendship groups — the glue that binds people together. We give a lot of ourselves, but also receive in return, and the likelihood of this happening only grows as we mature.

Celebrating long friendships

You can't make new old friends — it simply doesn't work that way. Meeting new people can be invigorating, but the subtle joy of sitting down with an old friend who shares a kind of shorthand with you offers a serenity and kinship that only comes from being long-time familiars.

Friendships go through their ups and downs — sometimes life, circumstances or even geography get in the way, leading to a sense of estrangement. But friendships can also, quite beautifully, come full circle, as it did for Anne-Marie, 56. 'When I was in my late thirties and early forties and my children were small, I found that many of my old friends didn't seem to be there for me anymore,' Anne-Marie explains. 'They were absorbed in their own things, or working hard, and dealing with increased responsibilities from parents, whereas I didn't have that to contend with. They had children at different times. One moved away.'

As a result, Anne-Marie says she often felt lonely, 'even when I had people to spend time with on a day-to-day basis. The quality of my relationships was not quite there, though. Conversations were stilted or too short, without much depth — I wasn't really getting what I needed. Slowly I met new people, mostly the parents of my children's friends.'

Now, in her mid-fifties, Anne-Marie has found that that many of her old friendships have come full circle. 'After a decade or more of intense parenting and careers, we have more time to spend together. There's something really special about being in each other's company now, just laughing over old jokes or stories we share. We mark out that time together,' she reflects.

'My newer friends have been around longer now too, of course, but it's those women I've known since I was in my early twenties or even younger who remind me of who I am and how far I've come.'

This sentiment was echoed by a number of older women — the sense of friendships being reinvigorated after various ups and downs.

But there were those, such as Vanessa, 61, who saw the same people, year in year out, and felt it made them who they are. 'My friend Elizabeth has always been in my life,' she says. 'Often our experiences have mirrored each other's in some way, almost at the same time, although we don't see each other more than a few times a year. We both got divorced around the same age, and as odd as it sounds, that was a real comfort. We speak on the phone a lot, or just check in with each other to see how the other is doing. With children the same age, we often experience similar milestones only months apart. When we took a trip recently to Turkey, we spent virtually the whole time in silence. But it wasn't a problem. With old friends, you often don't need to be "up" or anything more than what you are.'

Reassessing your relationships

If mid-life is a time for reassessing what really matters, then no subject deserves more scrutiny than our relationships, and whether or not they are still working for us. This doesn't mean walking away from people who don't meet our expectations — many of us would find that impossible to do, anyway — but re-establishing the rules of engagement so our relationships can continue forward positively.

One woman in her sixties I spoke with was married and worked part time, but says she has trouble asserting her needs with her children, who regularly call upon her for help with raising their own children. 'I love spending time with my grandchildren, and also helping out my son and daughter,' she explains, 'but there is a sense now that it's my time. I'd like the opportunity to explore this more, by finding out what other activities I'd like to do — beyond being a mother and a wife. Especially considering that I'm still healthy and active. I'd also like to travel, and hope I have the freedom to do so. It would be better if I could help out more sporadically or every once in a while, rather than on a regular, weekly basis. I'm not sure how this is going to pan out when I stop working altogether, as I think my children are expecting me to do more, not less.'

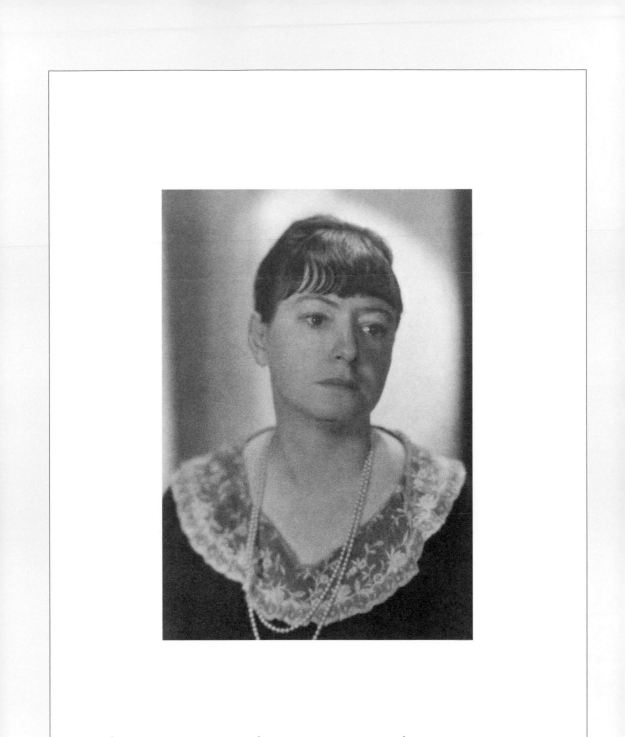

'ONE MORE DRINK AND I'LL BE UNDER THE HOST': DOROTHY PARKER,
FAMOUS WIT AND FOUNDING MEMBER OF THE ALGONQUIN ROUND TABLE

A number of women, ranging in age from their late fifties to early seventies, felt it was important to remain part of their family's lives, while also focusing at last on their own needs, at the risk of seeming 'selfish'. A woman in her seventies remarked, 'After years of child-rearing and looking after others, I think I have earned that right.' These feelings are mirrored in findings from an Ipsos Mackay social report on the recently retired, and a report by the company J. Walter Thompson Intelligence Group titled *The Elastic Generation*, which both focus on women in this age group.

Romantic partnerships can go through a renaissance or honeymoon period when the children leave home, but partners with differing views on how they'd like to spend their later years can also be the proverbial fly in the ointment, and even cause a marriage to come asunder in later life.

'Sometimes I think to myself, he has made a good first husband,' commented one woman in her fifties, of her husband of almost twenty years. 'He's been a great dad, but when the kids are grown and have moved out, I'm not sure I can see us remaining together. He's a lot less outgoing than I am, and has never been very interested in making friendships or exploring anything new, whereas these are things that are deeply important to and motivate me. I often wonder if I will meet someone who is more like-minded to share the next stage of my life with.'

Others feel that long-term relationships become challenging when they have made major life changes, but their partner has not shared the same journey — such as getting fit for the first time, or finding a new pastime — or vice versa. When one woman's partner discovered a new religion, for example, it upset the entire family dynamic and the way their relationship had operated up to that point, with her husband taking annual silent retreats of up to six weeks at a time and many weekends away, putting strain on the family and distancing him from daily life and relationships with his children and wife.

Independence is important, but most women prefer to exercise this without disrupting their families.

Charlotte Smith, 58, curator of the Darnell fashion collection and bestselling author, says growing older has changed the way she approaches many of her relationships. 'Growing older has made me wiser when it comes to people. Now I'm more purposeful in how I pick and choose those with whom I want to spend time,' explains Charlotte.

'I've stopped being polite about this, and although I would never be rude to anyone, I don't waste time building false friendships,' Charlotte says. 'I avoid, as much as possible, people who drain me of energy or fill me with negativity. There are so many positive people in the world I want to be surrounded by, I just don't have time for anyone who isn't.'

Sky News reader and author Jacinta Tynan, 49, says leaving an unhappy relationship was the hardest thing she has ever done, but now she has never been more at peace. 'When you tell people what's going on they always ask, why don't you just leave? But it's not that simple,' Jacinta reflects.

'Luckily I did have an income, so that gave me freedom and choices. But even then, it took me a long time to pluck up the courage. You keep hoping things will get better.'

On some level, at the start at least, Jacinta somehow believed that the relationship breakdown was all her fault. 'I spent many years of wasted time trying to "fix" it,' she recalls. 'But I don't regret that, because I will always know I gave it everything, and in time I'll be able to tell my boys that, so they'll know I didn't just give up.'

Like many women, Jacinta felt she should stay in the relationship for the sake of her two young boys.

'When you've got children, you feel like you owe it to them to stay in the relationship even if you're unhappy, to give them that stability. Lots of women do, because it's the hardest choice to make. I was prepared to suffer and compromise and give up my happiness,

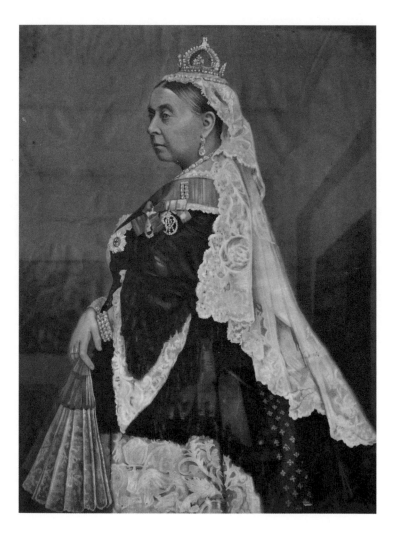

A GREAT LOVE STORY: QUEEN VICTORIA, WHOSE PRIVATE LETTERS
REVEAL HER SEXUAL ENTHUSIASM FOR HER HUSBAND, ALBERT

but in the end it became clear that it was impacting them as well. I knew then that I really had no choice but to go. I realised there was nothing more I could do to save the relationship or change the situation,' Jacinta explains.

'I had a lot of fear. It was a huge decision. But I knew the best thing I could do for myself and my boys was to leave our home and go and create a more peaceful life elsewhere, for all our sakes.'

This realisation was a clear turning point for Jacinta, who says she made it through to the other side with the help of a good therapist and daily meditation.

'A few years on, I feel really empowered that I had the courage to take that step,' she reflects. 'Gathering my two young children and leaving our home was the most frightening thing I'd ever done. It was very confronting logistically, emotionally and financially. But I also knew it was the only option. And now I can look back and feel really proud of myself. Like I can pull off anything.'

While she admits it's been tough going, the upsides have been profound. 'I am stronger than I knew,' says Jacinta. 'And I hope my boys can see that in me and gain strength themselves. That the very act of me stepping up will always remind them and reassure them that I will do anything for them, that I'm capable, and that my love for them will override everything. I've got their backs.'

Hitting the relationship reset button

If you're struggling with challenging relationships in your life, here are some general tips for making them more healthy and mature.

▸ **Set boundaries,** with friends, partners and co-workers — and especially children, parents and other family members. It can be a hard lesson to learn, but we absolutely do teach people how to treat us. If you're feeling like a doormat or emotional crutch for someone, address it. Teach people what's okay and not okay for you, and hold fast to your intentions for change.

Connection
& Sex

▸ **Beware of narcissists.** *Psychology Today* defines those with Narcissistic Personality Disorder as 'individuals who exhibit a lack of ability to empathise with others' and have 'an inflated sense of self-importance'. They are people who think the world revolves around them. You will never get what you need when operating in a relationship with a narcissist, so steer clear. If you don't have a choice (say, if you're related to one), strong boundaries will be more important than ever. Build up your reserves of emotional strength, and try not to expect too much from them; then, you won't be disappointed when they don't deliver the emotional goods.

▸ **Ditch co-dependency.** Relationships that are co-dependent aren't necessarily a bad thing, but they do operate under the assumption that neither member is a whole being on their own. Do the work that needs to be done on yourself first, rather than projecting your needs onto a partner, child or friend — or encouraging their sole reliance upon you, which is never great in the long run. And especially don't be a martyr ... this can be tedious for everyone around you.

▸ **Work out what's really important.** Some of us don't even know what it is we like to do in our spare time — we're so unused to having any. But a major part of wellbeing is finding out what we like to do for ourselves and pursuing individual goals — even if it's reading in bed with a bar of chocolate, or going for a long hike. There are ways to make this work within a relationship or family life, but first we need to define and create the space for it.

▸ **Say what you mean and mean what you say.** Passive aggression is irritating and doesn't always get the desired result. It's far better to be upfront and encourage open conversation with the people you care about. They will respect you for it even if, at first, the truth can be a bitter pill to swallow.

▸ **Reassess stale or toxic relationships.** There are times when the only solution is to walk away from a tricky friendship or even a family member. It's never done lightly, because it's hard to repair those sorts of connections once lost, but there comes a point where our own needs come first. If people consistently let you down, or make you feel used, upset or emotionally manipulated, it is only sensible to distance yourself.

▸ **Get help when you need it.** If you're really struggling to work out what you do and don't need from the relationships in your life, consider speaking with a psychologist or counsellor for some objectivity and practical tools (or a plan) to help you approach things differently. Help isn't just there for the big problems — it can also be about fine-tuning life to make it the very best it can be. You can't change other people's behaviour, but you can change your own reaction to it, and a counsellor can help you do that.

Long-term lovers

Good for you if your relationship is going great guns, and you and your partner still love each other deeply. Perhaps you're going through a golden period now that the children are grown and you have more time to spend with each other. The pressure of getting pregnant — or not getting pregnant — is finally over (hurrah!), and sex at this age can be more than just comforting: it can be downright liberating.

This is a time for celebrating how comfortable you feel with yourself and your partner. You know each other so intimately now, your likes and dislikes, your personal preferences, and it can be easy to jump straight to satisfying each other without all the trial and error of early love.

Except, what if the sex isn't so great? This can be confronting and upsetting, made worse by taboos or our own squeamishness when it comes to discussing it with our partner.

There is so much we can do to deepen (ahem, excuse the pun) that connection when life isn't so rosy in the bedroom. Over the next few pages, sex therapist Tracey Cox explains how.

How to age-proof your sex life

Q&A WITH TRACEY COX,

SEX AND RELATIONSHIPS EXPERT AND AUTHOR

▲

Tracey Cox, 57, is a popular television host, and author
of a forthcoming book about sex over 50. Often called upon for
her refreshingly honest advice on staying sexy and reinvigorating
relationships, she has a hands-on, taboo-free approach to getting
what you need under the sheets.

**What's your best advice for keeping the sexual spark alive
with our partners, or igniting one with someone new?**
Brush up on your sex skills. Technique is all-important as you
get older and in long-term relationships. It's not easy making love
to the same person for the rest of your life. Desire is dampened
by familiarity. It's imperative that your partner uses a technique
that works to bring you to orgasm. Without good technique,
you almost definitely won't climax or feel motivated to have sex.

If you're having sex with someone new, don't stress about your
body not looking like it did when you were twenty. Unless you've
gone for a much, much younger toy boy (go, girl!), their body isn't
going to be perfect either.

Sex is about what's happening on the inside, not the outside.
Close your eyes and focus on how you're feeling, not on how
you're looking.

A few of your best tips to age-proof your libido?

Use it or lose it. Remember that unless you're using penetrative sex toys, the only way to keep your genitals in good working order is to have regular sex.

The less often you have sex, the more likely it is that you'll find intercourse uncomfortable.

Be honest about what works for you, and keep your partner updated. Our bodies change as we age. Some bits need softer stimulation (penetrative sex needs to be slower and much gentler), while other bits might need a firmer touch — most women turn their vibrators up after they turn 50 or so, because things start to feel a little numb!

Sex before kids and after kids is different — things move around and our needs change. It's hard enough to keep up with your own body and what's happening, let alone expect your partner to somehow mind-read what you want and need now from sex.

The single, most important thing you can do to age-proof your libido and your sex life is to maintain an open, honest conversation with your partner about sex at every stage of your life.

There are solutions to every problem — make the effort to find them. Hormone replacement therapy, bioidentical hormones, testosterone supplements, fennel suppositories (yes, really — these are great for lubrication issues), estrogen pessaries, vaginal moisturisers, lube, 'bumpers' (squidgy things that he wears at the base of his penis during intercourse) to stop sex hurting — all work miracles to sort a whole host of problems. And if you're really keen, there's vaginal rejuvenation, electrode therapy for penises and a whole lot more. Don't be scared to ask for help, because there's plenty out there.

Use sex toys. Not just your vibrator for solo sex sessions, but in bed together. Sex toys are a cheap, instant way to introduce variety, and if you're having trouble tipping over to orgasm, they will help take the pressure off both of you.

Connection
& Sex

157

What could we do if we don't feel sexy anymore, or have a mismatched libido to our partner?

If you're not feeling sexy because you feel you don't conform to society's perception that you have to be young and thin to be happy, have a serious rethink. Sexy is an attitude, not a look or a size. If you're still convinced it is, get yourself off social media for a while or unfollow the Kardashians and follow some real, inspiring women who change the world through their intelligence and sheer force of personality (Michelle Obama, for instance).

Having said that, no one feels sexy if they're unfit and unhealthy. Feeling sexier might mean eating well, doing the right kind of exercise, or getting enough sleep. It might also mean making sex a priority in your life and taking responsibility to turn yourself on.

Think back to when you did feel sexy and liked having sex. What's different now to then? Pinpoint how you felt, what you did in bed, how your partner made you feel, and then do what you can to recreate those conditions.

For a mismatched libido, meet halfway. If you don't want intercourse, what about oral sex? If you don't want oral sex or any sex yourself, do you mind pleasuring your partner? At the very least, you are able to offer the physical intimacy of a cuddle.

Know what you want and need to be satisfied. And I'm talking both in, and out of, bed. If you need to relax first, don't be scared to ask for a massage. Or for them to do the dishes while you take a bath or shower.

Get your body clocks in sync. Is it really a case of mismatched libidos, or a morning person matched with a night-time one? If it is, take turns on the time of day you make love. On the weekend, try sex mid-morning, midday and mid-afternoon, rather than just morning or night.

'Sexy is an attitude, not a look or a size.'

▲

The
Power Age

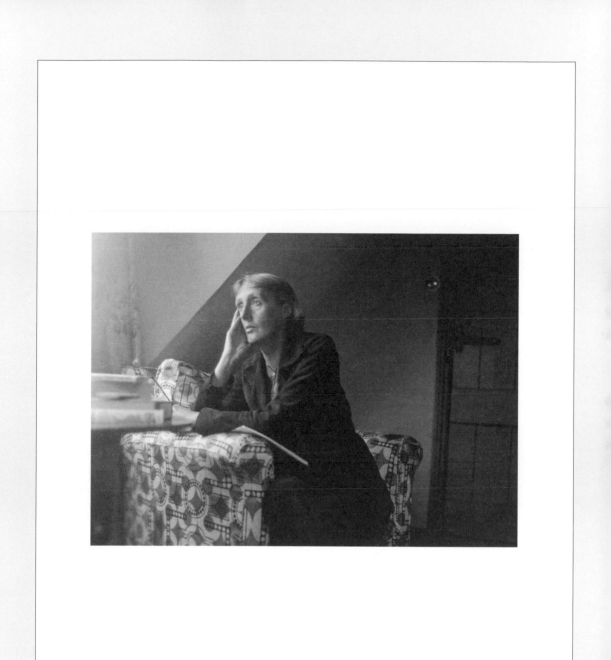

WRITER VIRGINIA WOOLF, PART OF THE
SEXUALLY EXPERIMENTAL BLOOMSBURY SET

**And lastly, you're clearly rocking your fifties, Tracey.
Do you have any tips for readers for doing the same at your
age and beyond?**

I drink loads of water — and I mean, loads! About 3 liters every
day. And I exercise, hard, a lot as well. I do an hour a day (five times
a week) of heavy weights (great for your bones and metabolism
and for maintaining muscle) and/or cardio (also with weights),
and balance that with 20 minutes of yoga in the afternoons.
It's not difficult to fit this in because I work from home. The yoga
I do online and in my office.

I've had Botox since I was about 30, but find I'm getting less
and less as the years go on. I don't like the frozen look anymore
(why was I ever fond of it, is more the question!). I haven't and
won't go down the filler route — I think it looks awful and like
you're desperately clinging on, rather than ageing gracefully.

I eat well, get lots of sleep and try to keep stress levels down
(only semi-successfully on that one). My one big, black mark is
drinking. I LOVE wine and drink far, far (far, far) too much.
I blame my husband: our favourite thing to do is plonk our
bottoms on the sofa, grab a bottle (or two) of wine and watch
a good box set. Yes, drinking is bad for your skin and your health
but we've got to have some vices or life would be very, very boring.
Perhaps because of where we live (in Notting Hill in London),
we eat out a lot. I love being surrounded by vibrant, young people
and like doing new things. Young people keep you feeling young.

If I had to summarise ageing happily and gracefully, I'd say drink
lots of water, lift heavy weights, eat well and sleep lots, but enjoy
life with everything else. Life's too short to deny yourself the things
you love. Feeling happy is what makes you look amazing; misery is
the most ageing thing there is.

Surround yourself with people you love and who make you feel
good about yourself. Get rid of anyone who doesn't (be ruthless).
Oh, and — of course — have lots and lots of sex!

**Tracey's top 3 things you can do right now
to revolutionise your sex life**

1. **Be realistic.** Stop comparing the sex you had when you were young and first met your partner to the sex you have now. Sex is different when you're older — in some ways challenging, but in lots of ways it's better than before. Adjust your expectations. Move the goal posts.

2. **Stop having 'comfort sex'.** You need stronger, lustier, more erotic turn-ons. Tap into more primal sex — explore fantasy, pornography, your darker side. All will reignite desire.

3. **Just do it.** Even if you're both gritting your teeth and could think of nothing worse, there is a strong argument for forcing yourselves to have some sort of sex on a regular basis. Desire isn't the only motivation for sex. Get yourselves back into a sex routine that will boost your libidos and remind you of how good sex can be.

THE LAST WORD

LUST FOR LIFE

▲

Midlife is usually a time of deep, long-term relationships. This is something to truly celebrate. We are often all the stronger for our friendships and marriages that have stood the test of time — they both lift us up and make us feel treasured in an otherwise uncertain world, and honouring them is important. The decades-long partnership and friendships, and relationships with older or fully grown children and parents ... they are all so precious and worth investing our time and energy in.

Relationships are not without challenges, but when we come through the other side we are often closer, and feel gratitude for the love and support they provide.

Nothing feels quite as good as being within our tribe, and connecting with those who matter.

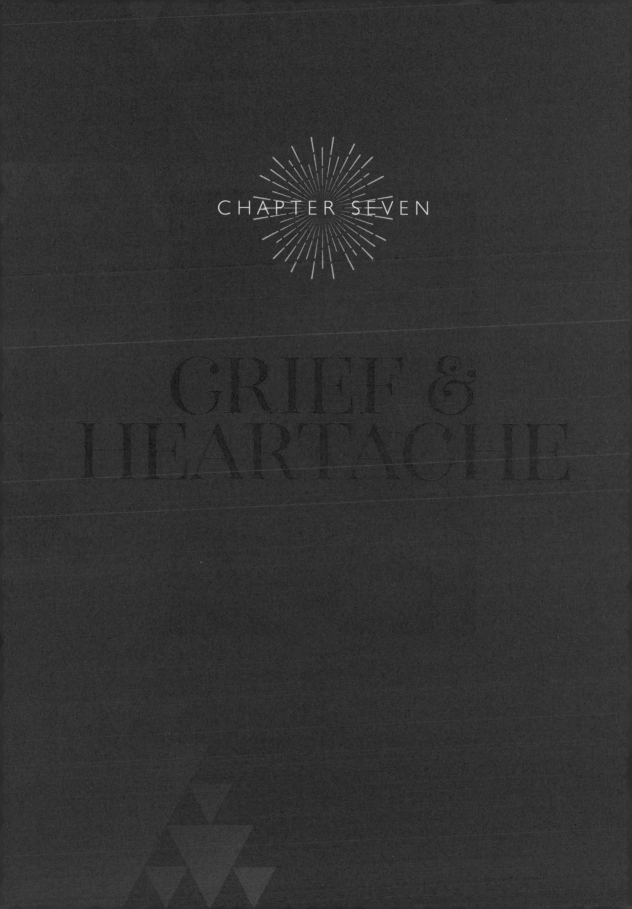

CHAPTER SEVEN

GRIEF & HEARTACHE

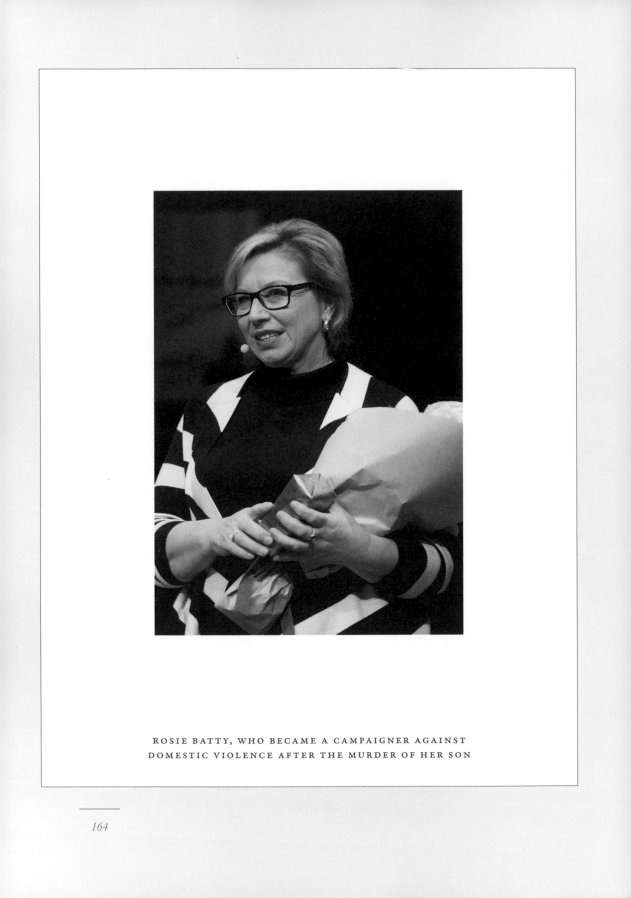

ROSIE BATTY, WHO BECAME A CAMPAIGNER AGAINST
DOMESTIC VIOLENCE AFTER THE MURDER OF HER SON

It's hard to talk about growing older without mentioning loss and grief, because none of us escapes this disco alive. What is most interesting and, well, human, is how we recover and return to our own sense of equilibrium. How we prove our mettle, time and time again, by asserting that we are incredible creatures, capable of such great capacity for strength and growth.

Through the accumulated pain of events such as miscarriage (which is such a common experience), parents dying, and even the death of a partner — as well as the sudden casualties of accident or illness along the way — loss is always heartbreaking, and always life-changing, whether it is experienced suddenly, or over an extended period of time. Divorce as well can be more traumatising than anyone expects, whether it occurs to you personally or within your greater family or social group.

No wonder it can sometimes feel life has turned a little sour.

But it is our hope and resilience that helps us continue when all else seems lost. It's what we take from our experiences that helps us understand life and, even, thrive.

Grief &
Heartache

———

Life is loss, but it's how we respond to it that counts

The following pages feature conversations with women who have endured different kinds of losses — the death of a partner, the loss of a friend, a health crisis, the loss of a baby — and what they learned. Each of these women, it has to be said, is now thriving, and radiates an enhanced degree of resilience, wisdom and empathy as a result of dealing with their painful experiences.

How to help others deal with loss

At some point or another, all of us will come in contact with friends and loved ones who are experiencing hardship or pain. So, how can you be a support and solace for them?

▸ **Make an effort.** Many people feel ashamed to admit they're struggling or to ask for help, but everyone needs a shoulder to lean on during difficult times. Even if, at first, they push you away, please keep trying. Stay in touch. Reach out often. Your efforts might feel mawkish or useless at times, but continue to simply be there for them, without judgement or expectation.

▸ **Listen.** Let your problems take a backseat in the relationship for a while, and don't make it all about you.

▸ **If you feel awkward, do something useful.** You could arrange for them to have a treatment or massage, or organise a network or group roster to make meals and help with childcare or hospital visits, for example.

▸ **Don't give up.** We all need love and compassion, and at some point it might be you who needs the help — that's the natural give and take of relationships and human connections.

▸ **Feel the love.**

We had twelve full years

INTERVIEW WITH FIONA INGLIS,
LITERARY AGENT

▲

Fiona Inglis, 58, represents *New York Times*-bestselling authors
Liane Moriarty and Markus Zusak at Curtis Brown. In 2015,
her husband John died of esophageal cancer, leaving Fiona with their
two sons, Will and Harry, who were nine and eleven at the time.
Here she shares her story of love and resilience.

Everyone called him Chook. We met through my colleague, Clair.
Her husband knew him and they tried to set us up a couple of times.
I thought he was gorgeous. He was so funny, he really made me
laugh. I was interested in him, but he paid no attention to me at all.

Then a few years later, in 2003, we threw a big party to celebrate
a management buyout at the agency. I was wearing a black satin
Max Mara suit, with a lacy top underneath and high heels (which
I never wear). Loads of clients and industry people came along,
and Clair invited Chook. The drinks party was meant to go from
6 pm to 8 pm, but by 10 pm I was walking around without my
heels, drinking champagne and smoking a cigar someone had given
me, because we'd bought the company, Curtis Brown. Chook and
I were standing talking on a little balcony off the main reception
area and he kissed me. I pulled away. 'You can't do that!' I said. 'All
these people are either staff or clients — this is really embarrassing.'

Grief &
Heartache

But he said, 'Don't worry, I'll sort this out.' He got a fork and banged it on a glass. 'I've got an announcement to make. I'd just like you all to know that Fiona and I have fallen in love, and we're going home together.' We were together from then on.

The party was in May, then I took a trip to London in September. I came home from the trip feeling really tired and jetlagged. I was 42 at the time, and I went to the doctor's because I thought something was wrong, and found out I was nearly 18 weeks' pregnant ... I was cooking, eating, not noticing I was putting on weight, and I wasn't ill — it was the happiest time of my life. He was watching a football match with his mates when I rang him to break the news, as we weren't living together at the time.

'Why are you crying?'

'Because I'm having a baby!'

'But ... isn't that the most wonderful news?'

I had no idea how he would react, but was thrilled and relieved that he, too, was ecstatic.

We found a house in December, and I was due the following March ... I was so happy being pregnant. Will was born ten days early. Then we had Harry 21 months later, after losing a baby in the middle due to miscarriage. We didn't waste time. We were lucky to have our two boys.

When Chook was diagnosed with cancer in September 2015, we asked the surgeon what the worst-case scenario was, and he said six months. We thought he'd be able to see our youngest son turn ten and our oldest son start high school, which was really important to Chook. But he was gone in six weeks.

Of course it was hard when he died. The funeral was a difficult day, but his friends came from all over the world, and the boys and I were reminded of how much he was loved.

The day Will started high school, the housemaster whisked him away to class and before I knew it I was left there standing in the quadrangle on my own. I felt utterly bereft. A friend of mine,

'The boys used to get upset when I cried, but I told them it's healthy to express emotion and shows how much we loved their dad.'

▲

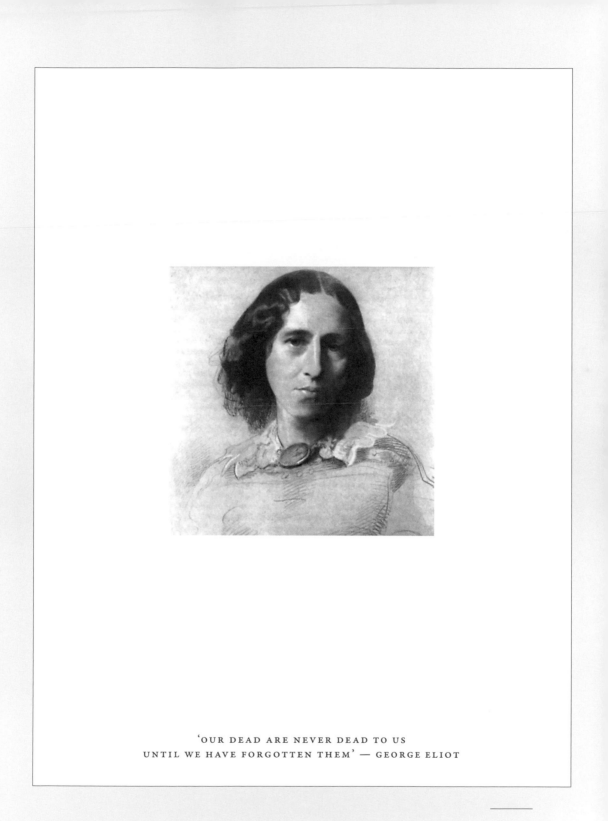

'OUR DEAD ARE NEVER DEAD TO US
UNTIL WE HAVE FORGOTTEN THEM' — GEORGE ELIOT

whose son was starting school at the same time, just came and wrapped herself around me. I don't know what I would have done without her. I think I would have melted into the floor.

It was devastating, but there are lots of positives about my story. I'm really close to my siblings and their spouses, and have a really good social group. I have great friends, and my work; I don't feel the absence of a partner in my life. We were together for twelve years, and packed so much into that time. I can't imagine anyone else being able to make me laugh as much. It doesn't feel like there's much space for someone else. Maybe one day, but I don't feel I'm missing out. I have everything I want.

The children and work are literally what get me up in the morning, but they also make me *want* to get up.

The boys used to get upset when I cried, but I told them it's healthy to express emotion and shows how much we loved their dad. Today's world is a confusing place for boys and young men, especially without the guiding hand of a father, but I hope I can help them to grow up as decent, caring human beings.

And I hope I am showing my boys that women can do whatever they set their minds to — they can run a business, and they can carry on in the face of adversity if they have support around them.

I will always miss her

INTERVIEW WITH LONE JACOBSEN,
DESIGN STORE MANAGER

▲

Danish-born Lone Jacobsen, 50, is a wife and mother of two.
Her best friend, Victoria, died suddenly while vacationing in Tenerife,
in Spain's Canary Islands, at the age of 48. Here Lone shares her
profound sense of loss.

I spoke to her on December 30, and found out she wasn't feeling well.
She said it was just a stomach bug, and she'd be fine. But she was dead
the following day. The doctors think she died of a brain aneurysm.

When her husband rang to tell me, I couldn't hold my body up. I
was absolutely devastated. It was the worst New Year's Eve ever.

My friend Victoria believed in Buddhism and life after death.
She definitely made me a more kind and giving person. She was
spiritual, and a dear friend — one of the kindest people in the world.

I loved her so much. As a person she was too much, sometimes
even for me! But she was wonderful, and I must have talked so
much about her — even after the period of acceptable grieving was
over. I could see people thought it was strange. I really didn't care. I
don't know if we were soulmates, but I often think about what she
meant to me — the world.

She is part of my story. How often do you meet someone like that?

When you can tell the story without crying, you have healed, and
I can tell it now with dry eyes. But I miss her. I will always miss her.

*'I must have
talked so much
about her — even
after the period of
acceptable grieving
was over.'*

▲

Grief &
Heartache

———

171

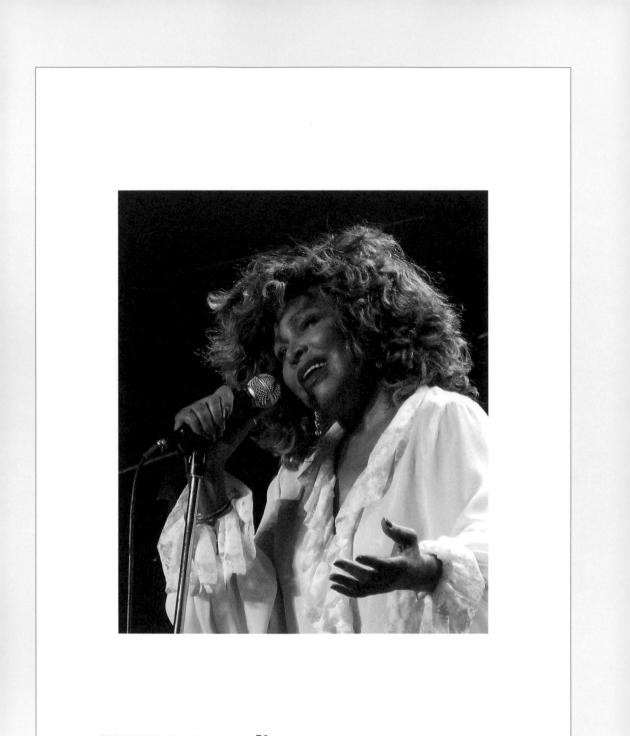

STRENGTH PERSONIFIED: 79-YEAR-OLD SOUL LEGEND TINA TURNER.
'PEOPLE THINK MY LIFE HAS BEEN TOUGH, BUT
I THINK IT'S BEEN A WONDERFUL JOURNEY'

Always hold onto hope —
because the darkness will not last forever

Q&A WITH HEATHER HAWKINS,
CANCER SURVIVOR AND MARATHON RUNNER

▲

Before being diagnosed with ovarian cancer,
Heather Hawkins, 54, was an everyday mom. She has
since run about twenty marathons and several
ultra-marathons, is an energetic fund-raiser for cancer
research, a regular speaker for charities, women's events,
sporting conferences and corporate and community
groups, and the author of a memoir, *Adventurous Spirit*.

How did your cancer diagnosis change your life?
Receiving my ovarian cancer diagnosis was a profoundly
confronting experience.

One Monday morning in February 2007 I was living my life
as a normal, busy working mom, by that afternoon I was fighting
hard just to keep going.

I am incredibly grateful for the skill of my surgeon and the care
of my oncologist, because I am one of the fortunate ones: I am a
survivor — one of the good statistics of this devastating disease.

Yes, it has changed me. Changed me profoundly. I am a
stronger, wiser, deeper version of my earlier self. I have a renewed
purpose to help others, particularly those affected by cancer.

Grief &
Heartache

I have a greater hunger to live life to the fullest every single day — and my adventurous spirit, which had lain dormant for so many years deep inside me, has been wonderfully reignited.

What's your advice for getting through the darkest of times and coming through the other side?

I have a little saying, 'The lowest points in life can actually be our turning points.'

When we're going through difficult and challenging times, it's perfectly natural to feel overwhelmed, saddened, broken. We all have a tipping point — but remember it's from this very point that we begin our journey back to being whole.

I've found that the first steps to navigating the darkness are actually small ones, and simply involve being kind to ourselves and recognising that our vulnerability and personal pain is not a sign of weakness, but an honest, brave reaction to the really tough stuff that we're facing right now.

To help in our recovery, it's important to focus on the things that we can control, and to learn to let go of the things we can't. Put a practical plan in place, stick with it, remain positive and always hold onto hope that there will be a way through.

Allow friends and family in to help share your pain.

Remember to look after yourself by eating healthily, getting additional rest, staying involved and connected in life (as much as you can cope with at the time). Listen to music and podcasts, write a journal (it's incredibly cathartic), and read books.

Exercise when you feel up to it — swim, walk, run, do yoga, pilates. It's a wonderful stress release, and I've found things always seem to be much more manageable when you're up and moving — and it has the added bonus of improving your fitness, too.

Remember that through this journey, the darkness will not last forever, you are much stronger than you think, and this may very well be the beginning of a whole, new amazing direction in life.

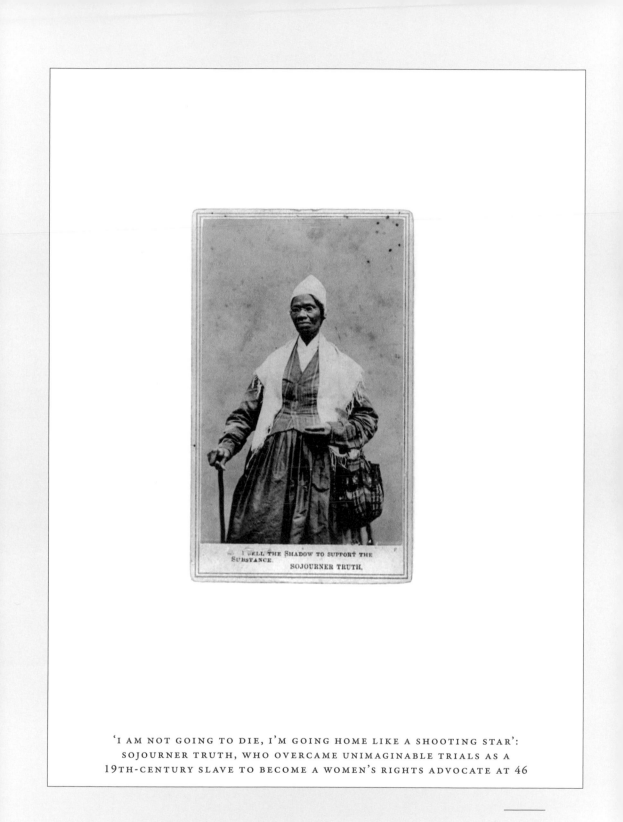

'I AM NOT GOING TO DIE, I'M GOING HOME LIKE A SHOOTING STAR':
SOJOURNER TRUTH, WHO OVERCAME UNIMAGINABLE TRIALS AS A
19TH-CENTURY SLAVE TO BECOME A WOMEN'S RIGHTS ADVOCATE AT 46

What do you look forward to?

As a child I remember my father saying, 'It's always important to have things to look forward to in life.'

As simple as it may sound, it's actually the most wonderful mantra to live by. It's liberating, empowering and fulfilling — because if we grant ourselves the permission to dream, to plan, and to get cracking to make these things a reality, then this will bring additional colour, opportunity and adventure to our lives.

What I'm looking forward to the most right now is my next ultra-marathon challenge, which is a 520-kilometer race, run over 10 days. It will be an opportunity to celebrate life, to push my physical and emotional boundaries,
and to grow!

And just as with every race that I do, I'll be running with the additional purpose of raising funds to improve the lives of youth facing cancer.

This means the world to me.

Leaning on your own
resourcefulness is empowering

INTERVIEW WITH REBECCA HUNTLEY,

SOCIAL RESEARCHER, AUTHOR AND HOST OF

'THE FULL CATASTROPHE' PODCAST

▲

After their daughter Sofia was born in 2008,
Rebecca Huntley, 47, and her engineer husband, Daniel,
immediately planned to have another baby, finally falling
pregnant a few years later. All seemed to be going well until
the five-month mark — when the unimaginable happened.

Tragically, it was then they found out that the baby had died
in Rebecca's womb. Rebecca went through a 12-hour labour to
deliver her stillborn child, then experienced numerous miscarriages
and rounds of IVF over the next four years before delivering
healthy twin girls, Stella and Sadie, who are now almost six.

'When you have to go through something that's a physical
process — for example, a long treatment like cancer, or operations
following a car accident, or anything where your body is going
through trauma — I think your brain creates a whole series of
walls around you while your body focuses on the healing it has to
do,' reflects Rebecca.

'It's not until your body has gone through that healing that you
can mentally process what has happened,' she adds.

Grief &
Heartache

'Even years later, I am still processing it emotionally. Only about 18 months after the stillbirth did I finally seek help. You could say it was too late by then, but I was so busy trying to heal physically. I was also going through IVF, and found it was crucial to have the support at that time.'

As a social researcher, Rebecca interviews people who have experienced a whole range of life experiences, and notes some telling patterns when it comes to miscarriage or stillbirth.

'In Australia, while there's been an increasing focus on mental health and destigmatising it, we still don't have those referrals and helpful pathways established for when people are going through grief and loss. I think I was handed a couple of brochures but, in the end, I sought treatment because a friend suggested it and I had the personal resources to do so.

'When bad things happen to people, we really need to make sure that their network and support is in full swing — for example, making sure that in a year's time after an ordeal, a GP talks to you about these things.'

After her stillbirth, Rebecca was fortunate that her IVF treatment was ultimately successful. While she herself experienced no problems connecting with her twins, she observes that some of that delayed grief and happiness can really impact upon the first year with your child: 'Many women and couples are so focused upon having another baby, when they finally do get the thing they've been wanting for so long and don't feel the immediate connection they expected, it can hit a lot harder and we see problems like postnatal depression.'

The process, she says, can also feel incredibly difficult for men. 'Generally, men are extremely poor at managing their own emotional health. They're not good at reaching out to their peers or friends. For example, when we lost the baby, Daniel told his colleagues and his friends about it, but not one person made special time to ask him about it or check he was okay.

'When bad things happen to people, we really need to make sure that their network and support is in full swing.'

▲

The
Power Age

'Everybody finds it really hard to talk about these things, but men in particular struggle, and I know Daniel found it hard with the twins because he was still processing his own grief. Without the peer networks, men find it difficult to handle the IVF process and miscarriages — and even if they Google "how to cope with miscarriage", much of the information out there is for or about women,' Rebecca explains.

'Our experience didn't affect his role as a father, but he didn't have the tools to deal with it. This is a personal, societal and systemic failure for men.'

For Rebecca, adversity uncovered a well of inner resourcefulness. 'I feel now that I do have a cast-iron stomach,' she says. 'There's not much that makes me feel *I couldn't really deal with that*. One of the problems I have with the term "resilience" is that it can sometimes be twisted to be an inditement. Sometimes life throws twists at people much worse than what I've dealt with, and I have wondered how they went on afterwards myself, but what it has taught me is immense resourcefulness. Some of this has been by dint of privilege, but it has built my sense of confidence in what I can cope with.'

Rebecca says she always knew, the whole way through, that if she didn't have another child, she would always regret it, and that even though she found the IVF process extremely trying, it also gave her the sense that it was worth it.

'When something is important, you really feel confidence to pursue it — almost single-mindedly, and without an enormous need for support. Weirdly, that gives you a level of confidence about the other things that happen in your life. I have an even greater trust in that now than I ever did.

'Looking back,' she says, 'it would have been nice not to feel I was going through something so big on my own — but I know now that I can, and that is very reassuring.'

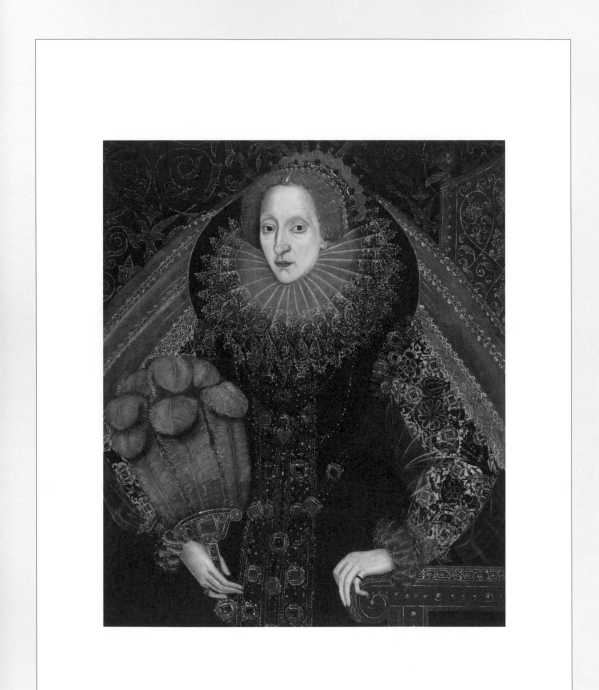

'I KNOW I HAVE BUT THE BODY OF A WEAK AND FEEBLE WOMAN,
BUT I HAVE THE HEART AND STOMACH OF A KING.' — ELIZABETH I

Rebecca's advice for healing the hurt after stillbirth or miscarriage

- **Seek help early,** however difficult this might feel.
- **Do your own research** about what you need, because medical practitioners are naturally conservative. Take charge of your own health and ask the sorts of questions that feel right to you.
- **Surround yourself with friends** and reach out to people who have had a similar experience. I was lucky enough to have one particular friend with almost the same IVF journey to walk with almost twice a week in the evenings — it was almost a kind of therapy for me.
- **Don't avoid the internet** as a source of information and support. You need to be selective, of course — there's so much information available out there, so work out which discussion sites are helpful, and where people are being supportive. I never posted online myself, but I read a lot on forums and worked out for myself the right way forward. The same goes for any trauma.
- **Focus on healing.** In the end, it may only be a very small handful of things that make you feel better, but if you can embed them into your routine, it really helps. For me, exercise therapy and being with a friend who understood me was critical.

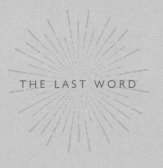

SOME FINAL TIPS ON SURVIVING GRIEF

▲

Dealing with loss or grief is never easy, but here are some simple strategies that can help you work through the process.

▶ **Surround yourself with your kin and community.** Remember that you are not alone. Reach out to others for help and support — sympathetic family or friends who love you and give life meaning. This can be a salve for your pain, and a source of solace that can help make sense of your own experiences and let you move forward.

▶ **Nurture yourself.** Grief is a huge physical and emotional burden. You'll feel better if you can do even small things each day to look after yourself, like exercising gently, eating well and getting enough sleep.

▶ **Stay active and engaged.** Not so busy that you don't have the opportunity to think about things, but busy enough to focus on something else for a while, or take a break from repetitive thoughts.

▶ **Don't struggle on alone.** This cannot be stressed strongly enough. If you're in trouble, seek professional help or reach out to an appropriate organisation. A counsellor or therapist can help you navigate this new terrain, and group meetings might help you feel less alone. Medication might even be a temporary fix to get you back on an even keel — but you'll never know if you don't seek help.

CHAPTER EIGHT

YOUR MONEY MATTERS

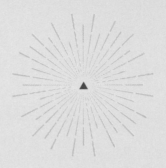

I t's true: money makes the world go around. And while it doesn't buy happiness, being fiscally fit — especially in mid to later life — provides a stable base that gives us the confidence and freedom of choice to pursue our dreams, whatever our age.

In many conversations with older women, having the funds to travel or even leave paid work for good are often top-of-mind. The fifties to seventies age bracket can look very different indeed for those with varying incomes or retirement savings, and while simplicity and focusing on what really matters is a common goal, many women also aspire to expand their horizons in this period. Money plays a significant part in that. Caring for ailing parents or boomerang kidults who have not yet established themselves in the world (or paying their ongoing expensive private school or university tuition fees) can drain otherwise-earmarked funds. The same goes for divorce, which can be catastrophic for women who have spent years out of the workforce due to child-rearing, and have missed out on contributing to their savings for later in life.

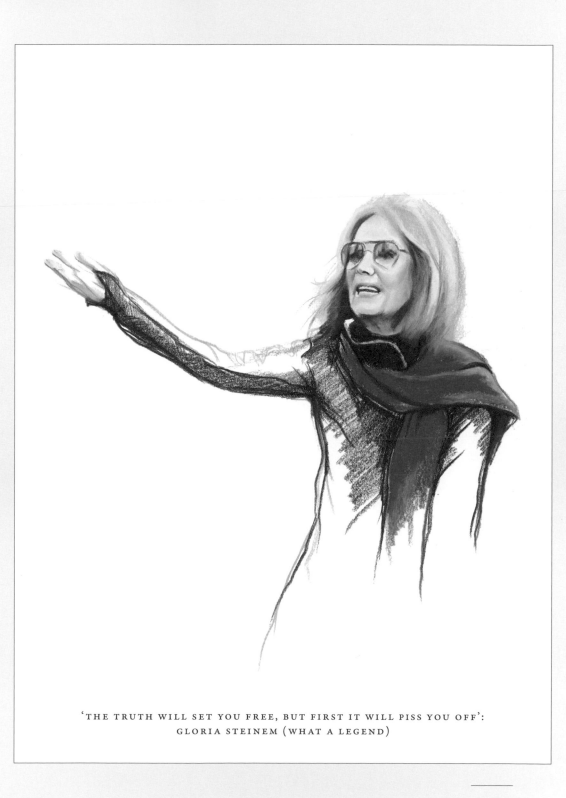

'THE TRUTH WILL SET YOU FREE, BUT FIRST IT WILL PISS YOU OFF':
GLORIA STEINEM (WHAT A LEGEND)

Some women I spoke to had been forced to continue working for a decade or more than they'd initially planned after the global financial crisis wiped out their savings, but for some of them at least, this has not been all bad. Meaningful employment provides a tremendous sense of purpose, and women of these generations are beginning to see — as men have in the preceding decades — the difficulties of redefining themselves after a stimulating and productive career that has commanded respect and admiration among their peers.

Retirement does not mean the same thing it once did. Rather than a period of 'winding down', some women feel they are just getting started, and relish finally having more time to be themselves. Many are active and healthy, and would like money so they can engage in experiences and interests they find enriching, or even push the boundaries of what they once thought possible.

Even if you do have enough money, this is a great time of life to make a difference and help others. Sofie, 57, administrates a charity she and her husband, an eye surgeon, set up to help cure relatively minor medical conditions that have a dramatic impact on the vision of people in developing countries. 'It really does make you feel good to help. We've worked hard for what we have, but have also been fortunate just by dint of birth and circumstance,' reflects Sofie.

'Travelling to these places and seeing the difference our money and the money we've raised makes is incredible,' she adds. 'I enjoy managing the funds and making sure they're well spent — every dollar matters and what would I spend it on here ... more art, more furniture? We don't need more vacations, and we have everything we need.'

Sofie remains largely unimpressed by wealth and its trappings, besides what it can do for those without it. She has also passed on this attitude to her children who, she says, despite growing up in affluent suburbs attending exclusive private schools, also seem remarkably unaffected or entitled. 'It's been valuable for our children, giving them a broader perspective and bigger sense of compassion for people than I think they would have had otherwise. They've seen the work we do and have been involved in it as well.'

But for many, philanthropy is seen as a 'would like to have', or the cream on top after a financially successful career.

Whether you are just gearing up for midlife and the different freedoms it promises, or you are fully into the swing of things already, it's a great time to review your finances, to give you the best possible base going forward.

Here are some simple tips for making the most of your dollars and ensuring you have the cash to do those things you'd most like to explore in your power age.

▸ **Contribute the maximum amount to your retirement savings.** In many countries, governments offer incentives to those who top up their retirement savings (superannuation, 401k) with voluntary payments. You can ask your employer to automatically deduct the additional amount from your salary before you get paid for the full tax breaks. What you don't see in the bank on payday, you really won't miss. Learn to live on what's left, and the savings will all add up.

▸ **Automatically divert 10 percent of your salary to savings each time you are paid.** Save little and save often — that's the simple trick to growing your savings. Cut down on frivolous expenses you can do without. It's oft-repeated, but those takeaway coffees every morning really do add up over time from our post-tax earnings.

▸ **Set up separate accounts for your disposable income.** You might not like keeping an eye on every dollar you spend, or following a strict budget each week (who does?), but try having automatic payments made into different accounts. This can be a great way to live within your means and feel flush at the same time. Do your research — many banks offer fee-free additional accounts, so it won't cost you anything. If eating out is important,

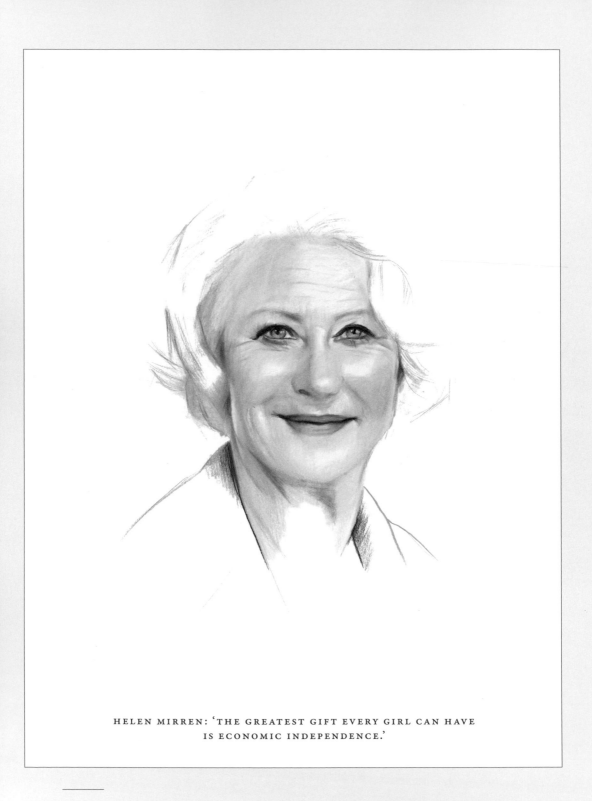

HELEN MIRREN: 'THE GREATEST GIFT EVERY GIRL CAN HAVE
IS ECONOMIC INDEPENDENCE.'

for example, set a weekly budget for yourself, you and your partner or your family as a whole, and have the money automatically transferred into this account. Same goes for regular salon visits, vacations or other 'necessities'. It can be very satisfying to watch your savings grow, but knowing that the money in these separate accounts is safe to spend at will can make you feel richer than Croesus. (Well, maybe not quite.)

▸ **Eliminate debt.** Now is the time to start consolidating your net worth, not racking up additional crushing debts. Can you live more simply and reduce your mortgage, or downsize and do away with it altogether? This needn't be as confronting as it sounds. While many people associate financial success with a big home and fancy car, the future will be more about apartment living and small homes anyway, according to town planners, governments and economists. Focus on what really matters — experiences and the people you love, not things. Not having a mortgage can mean the difference between staying in a job that makes you unhappy, or having the freedom to take a break and figure out what it is you'd like to do next. The debt-free life is a less anxious one.

▸ **Reduce credit card debt.** Some women are maxed out to the hilt. Sit down and take a cold, hard look at your spending habits, and assess your store and credit cards. Do you need them? Should you be saving up for treats, rather than splurging and paying later, with interest? Find a way to consolidate the debt, and set up automatic payments until they're fully paid off. This is tough love, but it might be time to destroy the cards altogether and start living within your means.

▸ **Monetise your talents.** For retired women who haven't actually earned enough savings for a comfortable retirement, how about taking up a part-time job or engaging in the gig economy? You could explore ways to make extra money from your hobbies — everyone has something to offer, whether it's garden design, sewing or practical business advice.

Ditch the rescue fantasy

ADVICE FROM SALLY LOANE,
DIRECTOR OF THE FINANCIAL SERVICES COUNCIL

▲

After 25 years as a journalist and nine years in the corporate sector, Sally Loane, 62, is CEO of the Financial Services Council, the peak industry organisation for fund managers, retail superannuation funds, advice licensees, life insurers and trustees in the financial services sector. Here she shares some tips for setting enough cash aside for a healthy retirement.

'Put as much money as you can into your retirement fund every week to top it up.'

▲

Financial independence not only gives us freedom, it also helps create resilience. Knowing that you're financially independent and in charge of your own economic present and future imparts enormous confidence and resilience.

Did you know that one of the fastest-growing groups of homeless people is women over the age of 55? The facts are not pretty. Young women consistently outperform their male counterparts in the classroom, yet go on to retire with around half as much in retirement savings. A new study in the city of Sydney revealed a shocking statistic: only one woman in 10 is confident she can rely on her savings in retirement. One in three women said if their relationship broke down, they would be at risk financially. Almost half said they were struggling or just getting along. These dreadful numbers are an indictment on our current system.

The
Power Age

Sally's tips for closing the gender retirement savings gap to feel more secure in later life

► Ask your boss for pay parity with male colleagues when you're both doing the same job. The gender wage gap starts for women in their twenties and widens to a chasm by the time they're fifty or sixty, having had time out of the workforce caring for children or elderly relatives (and of course it's still women who do this).

► Find an employer who offers female staff bonus financial advice sessions.

► Find a digital fund that offers change round-up features, which means every time you have a coffee or a beer and pay on a card, the virtual 'change' transfers into an investment fund. There are a few on the market now.

► Put as much money as you can every week (that takeaway coffee each day) into your retirement fund to top it up.

► Seek out a quality financial adviser. Research shows that women who do get financial advice are more likely to go on and own their home, mortgage-free.

► Think about whether you need life insurance if you're still relatively young (in your forties or fifties). You may want to opt out if you're in white collar work and you have no dependents. You can always opt in later on.

► Learn about money, and know where you can find information — from parents, trusted financial advisers, and apps specifically aimed at helping you be smart with your money.

► Women must ditch the rescue fantasy! No man, or woman, is going to rescue you with a huge pot of money. You won't win the Lottery, the government won't step in and save you, so stop thinking there is anyone or anything other than yourself that will help you become financially independent.

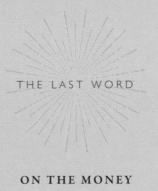

THE LAST WORD

ON THE MONEY

▲

Pass on good money habits to your kids, especially your daughters. This will not only help them, it will help your own finances in the long term because you won't need to be constantly bailing them out as adults.

And be smart: don't spend blindly or without any idea about the impact your choices have on your financial health. Research investments thoroughly, save for a rainy day and take control of your money.

As the sublime actress Helen Mirren once said, 'The greatest gift every girl can have is economic independence.'

Make that your motto.

CHAPTER NINE

PAY IT
FORWARD

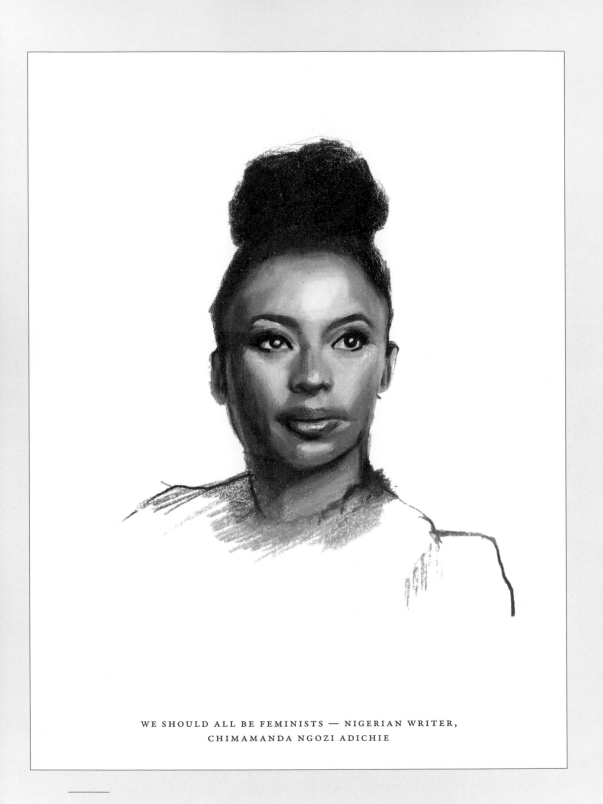

WE SHOULD ALL BE FEMINISTS — NIGERIAN WRITER,
CHIMAMANDA NGOZI ADICHIE

T here is a saying that if you want to feel better, do something for yourself. But if you want to feel fulfilled, do something for someone else. Of course, grown women understand the concept of sacrificing our own needs for others, sometimes to the point of there being little left for ourselves. But we also understand the intrinsic value of giving.

Scientific research backs this up. Being generous is *really* good for you. It releases endorphins into your system, similar to when you exercise. The 'love hormone' oxytocin floods your body, making you feel more connected with others, and lowering your stress levels in general. Do good in your own small microcosm, and it has a wonderful, ripple-outwards effect, spreading to those you love and beyond. Which is why philanthropists find giving and doing good such a high.

Who knew? Paying it forward can be as addictive as a drug.

But why 'indulge' in being altruistic now, even if you haven't previously felt the headspace to do so? Well, because you might have more time on your hands, or have accumulated more experience

Pay It
Forward

———

195

and wisdom at this point in your life which you're able to share. Maybe your cup runneth over, as it were, and you've developed a better sense of social and spiritual connectedness. Either way, many women do find that, after a certain point in their lives, helping others is far more satisfying than helping themselves.

You don't need to make big, flashy or time-intensive gestures like donating huge sums of money, or volunteering in a soup kitchen every weekend. Simple deeds make a powerful impact. Maybe it's offering to look after a friend or neighbour's children for the evening so they can go out for dinner or a weekend away; maybe it's letting someone slip into your lane in bumper-to-bumper traffic; or maybe it's offering to fetch your stressed-out colleague some lunch when they're chained to their desk. Buy a homeless person a meal, or drop off a thoughtful gift to a friend *just because*. Smile at strangers. Forgive those who have hurt you.

Trying to feel better yourself is not *why* to commit spontaneous acts of goodwill, but you'll certainly reap the rewards later.

As you will see from the women profiled in this chapter, there are myriad causes and a million ways to help out. You can incorporate making a difference into your daily life so that you're helping someone, while also supporting yourself and doing what you love.

So much confidence comes from helping others

INTERVIEW WITH MAGGIE BEER, COOK, RESTAURATEUR, FARMER, BUSINESSWOMAN, TELEVISION HOST AND AUTHOR

▲

Beloved culinary icon, cookbook author and television presenter Maggie Beer has always understood the value and joy of honest good food. Now she has made it her mission to improve the quality of life of elderly people in a meaningful, practical way — every single day. The rewards have been immense.

In 2010, after being named Senior Australian of the Year for her many years as a passionate and enthusiastic food educator, Maggie was inundated with around 900 speaking engagement offers, and wondered how she could really make the most difference to people's lives.

'I spoke at an event to a thousand CEOs of aged care facilities, and that's when my own life really changed — though it took a while for the journey to unfold,' Maggie explains.

'I did a lot of research on the state of the food being offered in aged care homes, and what I found was both great and terrible. The terrible was not to be accepted, and the great to be celebrated and used as benchmarks. I gathered a team of people around me with the right skills and strategies to help.'

Pay It
Forward

And so, in 2014, The Maggie Beer Foundation came into being, to improve food experiences for older people, particularly those living in aged care homes.

As well as engaging CEOs, its focus, says Maggie, 'is upon providing practical cooking advice and knowledge about the nutritional value of food to the kitchen staff in homes. We do this through masterclasses that bring together 30 cooks and chefs at a time, and draw on expertise to give them the skills, ideas, passion and respect they deserve so they can make food that counts for residents — food that they can actually enjoy.'

The Foundation runs on the 'smell of an oily rag' according to Maggie, but is making a difference thanks to its team of highly committed people and the passion of its founder.

Maggie has made it her personal mission to link the latest research on how the food we eat can impact brain health, with her innate knowledge of what good food can do for a person's emotional wellbeing.

'What I learned is that you have to get *everyone* behind you in a home,' explains Maggie.

'The word *facility* — the F word — should never be used because it's where people live; it's their *home*,' she points out.

'Cooks and chefs are working so hard and they want to make a difference. They so deserve to be given the ability to do this, and then be given the respect they deserve. There has been so much feedback from these masterclasses from the cooks and chefs, telling us it's changed the lives of those they look after by making them happier and healthier.'

Not satisfied with the impact she was having through the Foundation's masterclasses and other activities, the Foundation is on the cusp of setting up an online training program so its message can spread to nursing homes that haven't been involved, and other organisations that provide food to the elderly, to nurture more people at the end of their lives with good food.

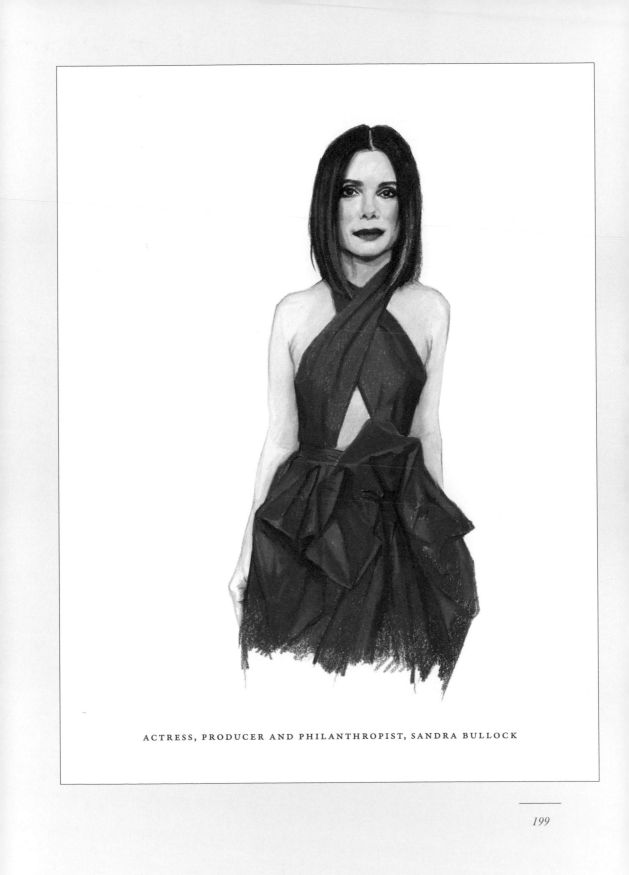

ACTRESS, PRODUCER AND PHILANTHROPIST, SANDRA BULLOCK

'Success has come from loving what I do, believing in it, and having a mind that needs to see ideas through,' says Maggie.

'My advice to anyone looking to make a difference themselves is to take it seriously. Go do something for someone else and see how it makes you feel — there's nothing like it for giving meaning to your life,' she suggests.

'Find a cause that's going to resonate with you personally, because we all need to be connected and have purpose over and above our own lives. It's a given that you need to look after yourself first, and women in general are not good at that — but it's a two-way street: so much confidence comes from helping others.'

Maggie's enthusiasm shows no signs of waning.

'This has been the most amazing and rewarding thing I've ever done in my life — I think I'll be forever doing it! Soon I'll be 75, and have promised my husband I'll slow down. By that I mean, not working 70 hours per week.

'But I get so much energy from ideas, people, food, family and music. I also live in a beautiful place in the country with people I love, and in a good community.

'For me, age is just a state of mind — not a number.'

'Go do something for someone else and see how it makes you feel — there's nothing like it for giving meaning to your life.'

▲

Passion and clear vision
can overcome all obstacles

▲

When dreams turn to dust, a higher vision sometimes arises,
as Kit Willow's story below shows. At only 23 years of age,
Kit started her eponymous fashion label, Willow, long celebrated
for its impeccable tailoring and feminine suiting, as well as its elegant
lingerie-as-outerwear aesthetic. Everything appeared to be going
well, until events took an unexpected turn. Here we see how
'doing good' can change things for the better.

After taking on an angel investor as an equity partner, the business continued operating successfully until Kit's angel investor sold his shares, with Kit's consent, to a fashion group. Kit was in equity partnership with the new group for 18 months — before being ousted from the company she had so passionately built from scratch.

The experience was utterly heartbreaking.

After a period of wondering whether to move to a seaside town and become a yoga instructor, she started her second company, kitX, changing the focus of her new fashion label to a sustainable one, to bring about a positive change and pay it forward for the environment. In hindsight, she can see that the shift has been worthwhile on so many levels.

Pay It
Forward

201

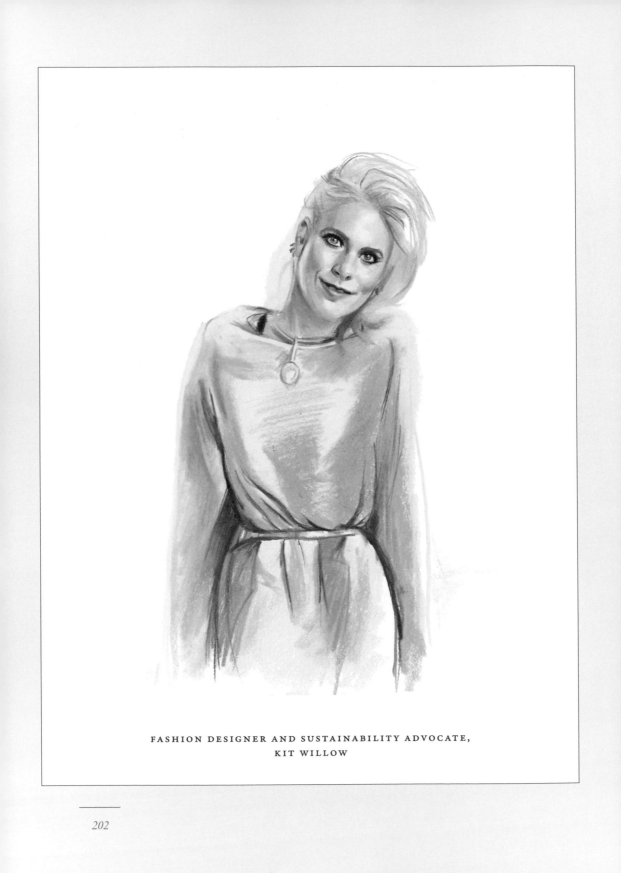

FASHION DESIGNER AND SUSTAINABILITY ADVOCATE,
KIT WILLOW

'In the period after Willow disappearing, I had a good while to reflect,' Kit muses. She did some deep research into the fashion industry, and what she discovered shocked her.

'The fashion industry is second only to oil in its impact on the environment,' she says.

'It starts at dirt level with the pesticides and chemicals they use, and it wastes such enormous amounts of water through the production process. And man-made fibers such as polyester give off toxic chemicals that don't ever properly break down when they're put in landfill. You think you're doing good when you give your old clothes to charity shops, but a lot of it ends up in landfills. About 13 trillion tonnes per year in America alone.'

Up until that point Kit had assumed, like many of us, that by recycling and paying attention to Willow's packaging that she was making a positive impact. It wasn't until she was invited by the Climate Council to learn more that she began to understand how dire the situation for fast fashion really is.

'The fashion industry needs a complete shake-up. It's a broken system,' explains Kit. 'The world simply can't sustain fast fashion and the impact it has upon the planet — we don't have enough resources, and when you pair it with the population boom, you realise that our ecosystem is under a huge amount of pressure.

'We are at a critical point in history. If we don't stop carbon emissions, the temperatures will keep increasing and the lungs of the earth will die — there will literally be no natural living forest left by the year 2100. No seafood or agriculture, and clean drinking water will be in short supply. It's frightening.'

Alarmed into action, Kit found herself questioning the status quo. 'I'm trying to work out a new way by asking, *What's the new model?*' she explains.

'I want to cut down on the number of styles I'm developing, and make sure that they don't need to be marked-down at the end of each season, or turned over so rapidly. I have access to this privileged

'The world simply can't sustain fast fashion and the impact it has upon the planet — we don't have enough resources.'

▲

information through the Climate Council, and it's fascinating to be involved in — I'm excited by the prospect of what can be achieved.'

For potential business owners who want to pay it forward and make a difference, Kit offers the following advice: 'It's not for the faint-hearted. It's very hard, but if you're passionate and have a clear vision, then you can overcome all obstacles. Being positive and a realist is really critical.'

Following a passion helps, too.

'I love what I do in designing and creating fashion — I've always been obsessed with it,' says Kit.

'It's not a large percentage of what I do every day, but that feeling of being in fittings and draping and working with fabric is such a great high ... I think women are amazing, especially working mothers. I want to make them feel empowered and strong — that's always been a driving force for me.'

True altruism is doing something for others even when it doesn't benefit you. Be generous.

Lifting other women up

INTERVIEW WITH CATHERINE FOX,
AWARD-WINNING JOURNALIST AND AUTHOR

▲

The idea that women function poorly in positions of power is deeply embedded within our society, and can be traced back to ancient Greece and Rome. One really powerful way to give back and feel good about yourself is to mentor and support other women. Catherine Fox, 60, author of *Stop Fixing Women* and co-author of *Women Kind*, explains how it can make the world a better place.

Women are actually wonderful mentors. The idea of the Queen Bee, or women turning on each other — especially in the workplace — is a story we're told to keep us away from positions of power, but there is actually very little evidence for it.

Women self-select into support groups all the time. Which absolutely contradicts the idea that we're somehow not good at it. The #MeToo and #celebratingwomen campaigns have been all about this; women coming together and backing each other up to take a stand. They're not making this stuff up. It's great to see women working together and calling injustices out. Importantly, the emphasis is on doing things collectively.

By and large, women often do have a fantastic network of friends, colleagues, other women and people they've met through all parts of their life who help and support them. There is a huge

Pay It
Forward

'There is a huge
sense of purpose and
value that comes
from supporting
others, particularly
younger women.'

▲

sense of purpose and value that comes from supporting others, particularly younger women. Women have been doing it forever, but it would be great to see more of it. I'm not talking about women being faulty in some way or needing to be fixed — women have been on the margins of power for too long, battling stereotypes and systemic bias, and they're often penalised if they don't conform to classic stereotypes of caring and empathy. But this is not a legacy of gender, it's one of power.

There were a number of women in the first administration of U.S. president Barack Obama who had an idea for supporting other women. They decided to back each other up in meetings, so there wasn't a chance for them to be interrupted or their contributions ignored. They called this idea 'amplification', and congratulated each other publicly when they did good work. Women stepping up *definitely* has an effect. It's life sustaining.

It's incredibly important for everyone to seek advice and get inspired by other people we can see doing well, but this doesn't necessarily have to be someone more senior than you. You can get real assistance and value by having a peer mentoring system, which is also useful.

I'm an optimist. I think things are changing. Partly through social media, which is the last thing we've expected. I casually mentor people, but have also personally benefited from other women stepping up to help me. Often as mentor, the most important role is to offer a different perspective, and simply ask: *Have you thought about this?* Because when you're immersed in the daily grind it's not always clear.

Being able to do that for someone else is enormously fulfilling. I have three daughters and try to help them in that way all the time. It's about getting to know someone, understanding them and encouraging them to think differently.

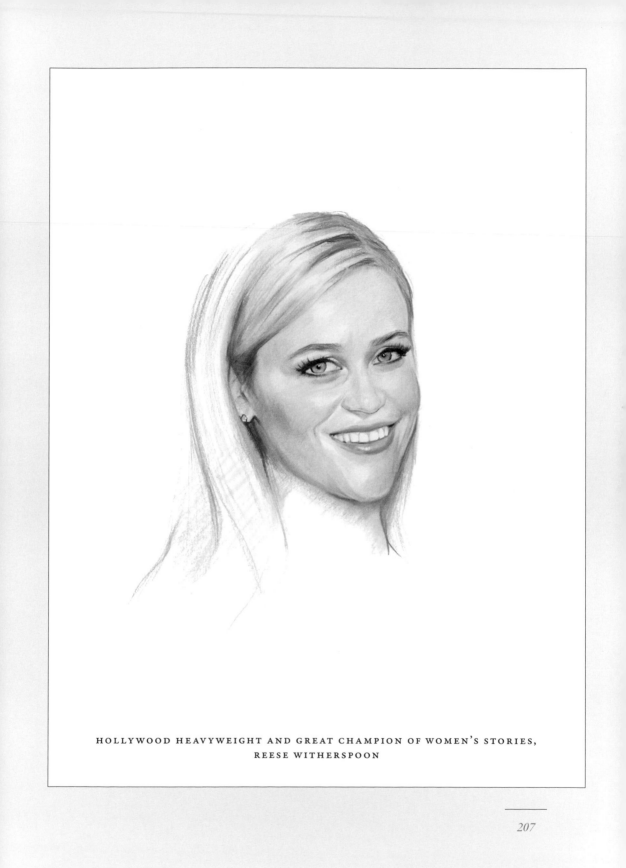

HOLLYWOOD HEAVYWEIGHT AND GREAT CHAMPION OF WOMEN'S STORIES,
REESE WITHERSPOON

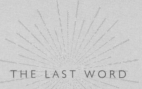

THE LAST WORD

THERE'S SO MUCH YOU CAN DO

▲

If you want to get out there and make a difference, but are finding it difficult to decide where to start, work out what really matters to you. Is it caring for children, or animal welfare, for example? Or is it research into preventing diseases such as cancer or early-onset Alzheimer's? If you care about a cause, you'll be more invested in it, and more likely to commit your time, money and energy.

Many charities and community organisations need something more than funds: they need time and expertise to do their best work and spread their message. It's worth having a really good think about your background, skills and the ways in which you might be able to share those with an organisation that matters to you.

It's also a good idea to look around your community and simply ask yourself, who needs the most help? If you can't decide, just start with something. Making even a small contribution is always better than doing nothing.

If you have any sort of platform or influence, try using it to help raise awareness of their good works, and be generous. Remember, your health and happiness are the side benefit.

CHAPTER TEN

CELEBRATE
YOU!

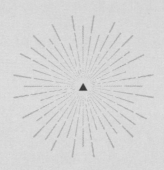

As fashion designer Diane von Furstenberg says in her autobiography, *The Woman I Wanted to Be*: 'Living also means ageing. The good thing about ageing is that you have a past, a history. If you like your past and stand by it, then you know you have lived fully and learned from your life.'

We've heard from a number of savvy, inspiring older women throughout this book, but now it's time to consider what your own power age looks like. Here you'll find some final suggestions for how to make it feel better than ever.

Stop caring what people think

Keep a healthy distance between yourself and anyone who puts you down or makes you feel bad about yourself. It's said nobody can *make* us feel anything, but we can certainly remove ourselves from the situations and triggers that conspire to make us feel rubbish. Nothing says grown-up like Rising Above. This could be from the friend who gives you the guilts because you don't call often enough, to the partner who says, 'Oh — you're wearing *that*?' and frowns until you change. It's high noon to march to the beat of your own drum because, well, if not now, then when?

There's a saying that roughly a third of the people you meet in life are going to realise how great you are, another third will actively dislike you, and the last third will be coolly indifferent to your charms. Operate on the assumption that it's true, and you may find it quite liberating. You might even find that if you locate your inner fabulousness on a daily basis, more than a third of the people in your life will cherish you and value you for the precious gem that you are.

Be yourself

We humans are extraordinary beings. We all have our numerous faults, weaknesses and blind spots, but most of us are just trying to make our way in the world in the best way we know how, and trying to treat others the way we'd like to be treated ourselves. Where youth knows so much with solid certainty, wisdom reveals that all, in truth, is shifting shades of grey.

It's reassuring then that, in our later decades, we can finally start accepting our unique qualities, along with our foibles. Because experience gives you one thing above all else: a broader perspective on life and those around you. It also wises you up to the truth that parts of your personality might have become quite fixed over time. It's always possible to change them, but would you really want to? Aren't all our qualities or faults just one side of the coin?

Rather than labelling your qualities as 'good' or 'bad', think in terms of balance. Are you out of whack, or are you just right? Is your bleeding heart also the source of your compassion? Is your severity actually part of your strength?

The thing about growing older is that you begin to fear *not* being yourself, more than you care about how other people will behave when you are. Just like demurring from what we really want to say or do makes us feel somehow *less than*, authenticity — when practised often — becomes an innate quality deep inside us, which we exhibit every day through the choices we make and the things we do.

The woman who is utterly true to herself glows from within. She will say, *No, I'm not fine*, when something awful happens. She will tell you what she really thinks instead of hiding her truth, and she will show you her open, beating heart — scars and all. It may be a messy or raw experience, and it may make other people feel uncomfortable, but it's real. And real is a thing of beauty. Embrace it.

Perfect your ageless chat

Avoid Smug Married dinner party conversations and other yawn-fests. This means property market discussions (gah! The worst!), the 'youth of today' or how you just don't get X. Try switching the conversation to the latest scientific research you just heard about, your dream of high-altitude hiking in Peru or the new novel you're reading. Artificial intelligence? Bungy jumping at eighty ... Why not? And screw the old adage about no religion, sex or politics at the dinner table — they're the best kinds of subjects, which will leave you arguing well into the wee hours. Nothing gets the blood up (or brings a lively flush to the face) like a little lively, conversational dispute.

Realise that perhaps the best way to perfect your ageless chat is to first experience something new. This doesn't have to mean jetting off to India for a shift in perspective. It can simply be through watching or reading something unusual, like attending a local Iranian film festival, or swapping your favourite genre fiction for a challenging non-fiction book about evolution, technology or the memoir of a person who has lived an interesting life very different to your own.

Talk about ideas, not people. Swap gossip in favour of learning something new that will inspire you to think differently. Ask the off-piste questions, and you might be surprised by the answers.

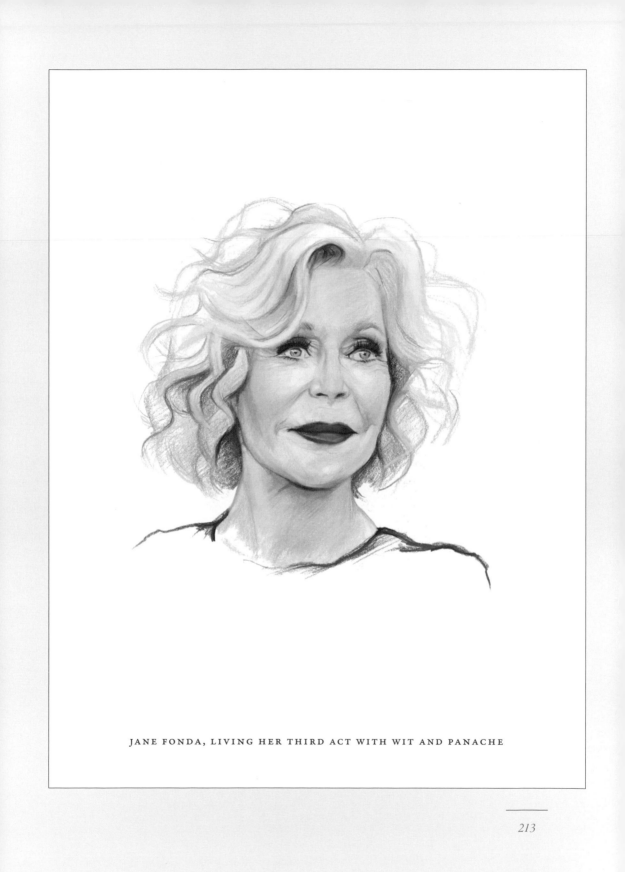

JANE FONDA, LIVING HER THIRD ACT WITH WIT AND PANACHE

And if your current set of friends just aren't interested in getting out of their conversational rut, find some new ones. Which brings us to ...

Make new friends

Good friends who love, support and make you laugh will always keep you young, but hanging out with the same people day in, day out is ossifying as you age.

Are you the sort of person who feels awkward at parties, especially when there are a lot of younger people in the room or those you don't know? Rise above it. Set yourself the challenge of befriending at least one new person a year, and incorporating them into your life, and your existing group of friends. It could be through work, or a loosely based social circle like your book group or gym class.

Ignore age — you wouldn't want someone to dismiss you for being the age you are, so don't do it to others. Have friends of a gloriously wide spectrum in both years and mindset. This is a prescription for staying open, informed and youthful at heart, and it will make you wonderfully adaptable to many new situations.

How to be authentic

► A very small first step, but when asked if you enjoyed your (too cold, oversalted) meal, be honest. Say it with a smile, but realise that the world will not stop spinning on its axis if you complain. We women are so used to smoothing things over, ever playing the diplomat, but sometimes you just have to call it when things are not up to scratch.

► Don't be afraid to speak your mind in the boardroom or other work situations. There are many ways to get your point across without pissing people off. Those who complain and whine without making any effort to change the status quo are the worst.

- Buy and wear clothes that will bring you joy every time you wear them, rather than conforming to what you think you should look like, or what everyone else in your age or social group seems to be wearing. Mix it up. Be bold.
- Ditto with your travel and vacations. Challenge yourself, doing only those things that hit you squarely in the solar plexus and make you feel right.
- Take regular stock of what you spend most of your time doing. Do your days generally make you happy, or does the grind of your everyday existence feel, well, like a bit of a grind? Life is not meant to be a constant roller-coaster of excitement, but if you're feeling dissatisfied, something needs to change, because the way we spend our days is, after all, the way we spend our life.
- Write a list of the things you enjoy doing most. Perhaps it's walking in nature, attending a yoga class or catching up with old friends for dinner and drinks. Perhaps it's cuddling up in bed with your partner or playing with your grandkids. Try making more time for life's pleasures, and avoid too many tasks that make you feel crotchety and 'over it', or at least balance them out with more moments of pure, indulgent joy.
- Fill your bucket by looking after yourself and staying healthy. A weekend spent catching up on sleep or singing karaoke with a group of friends until the wee hours can be just as restorative as a lengthy trip to the skin clinic or hairdresser. There's absolutely nothing shameful about enhancing your looks or working them to your best advantage, but nothing replaces that inner smile of a woman whose life is well-lived. Within as without.

Celebrate
You!

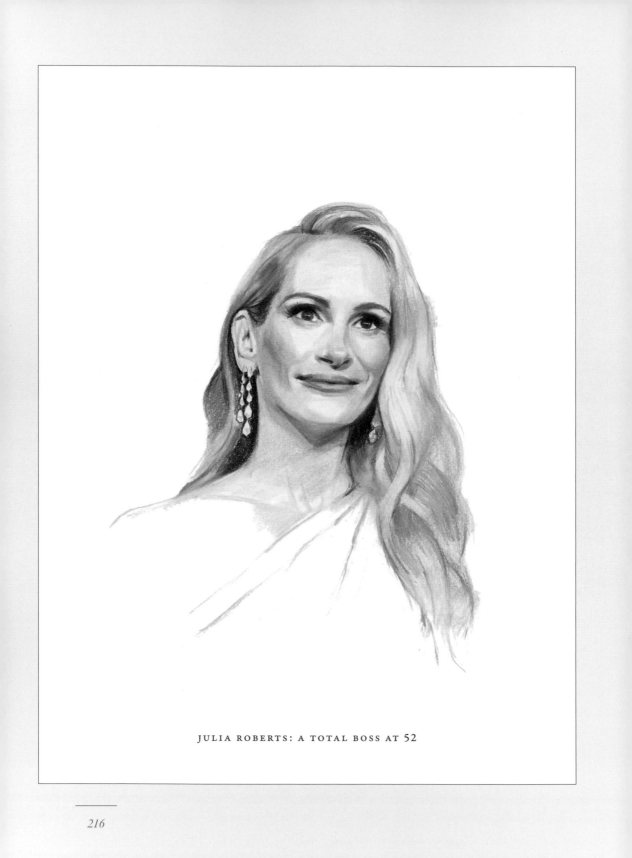

JULIA ROBERTS: A TOTAL BOSS AT 52

Nordic societies have a thing or two to teach us, in this respect. Particularly the Danes. Statistically, every Dane is a member of four or more social groups. No matter how shy or quiet you are, just being a part of a group creates bonds that make us feel happier and better adjusted. Also more able to cope with the challenges life sometimes throws at us.

How many social groups are you part of? Are there others you could join?

Embrace your vintage

So much about loving your age is learning to be comfortable with the process and embracing the positives. If you look and feel the very best you can, then that's what it's all about: not looking younger, just looking *great* — no matter what age you are.

Some women clearly aren't comfortable with it. Canadian gossip columnist Lainey often refers to 'L.A. Face' — that frozen, caught-in-a-wind-tunnel look, thanks to facelifts, too many Botox treatments, skin resurfacing and collagen injections which seem to make everyone look, rather boringly, the same. It's also all a bit, well … porny. Have you noticed how cosmetic enhancements have become the norm? You're not alone. The sort of pouts that used to only be seen on the cover of X-rated videos are now everywhere. Somewhere between Jocelyn Wildenstein (aka 'Catwoman') and the rise of the Kardashians, it became acceptable, and it feels slightly bonkers if we're all down with it.

You are only as old as you feel: say it loud, say it proud. It's true.

Celebrate
You!

Stay staunch to yourself

INTERVIEW WITH YUMI STYNES,
JOURNALIST AND RADIO HOST

▲

The author of two feminist cookbooks (*The Zero F*cks Cookbook* and *Zero Fucks: Endless Summer*), Yumi Stynes, 44, also hosts the award-winning ABC podcast, 'Ladies, We Need to Talk'. Covering topics like ageing, menopause, periods and female adultery, she developed the series with co-producer Claudine Ryan to break down taboos and open up conversations among women.

Yumi isn't afraid to speak her truth. 'I've never really cared about what people think,' she says.

Growing up in a small town with a Japanese mother and an Australian father, she was always aware of being the 'other'.

'We weren't mistreated or disrespected, but we were clearly "that Asian family". I had no anonymity. People would literally stop in the supermarket and stare at my mother when she shopped — they were so unused to an Asian face.'

Because of the way she looked, Yumi says she could never really blend in, 'so I just shrugged and got on with it. Both my parents were terrific influences in that way — my dad was never even faintly interested in the opinions of others, and my mother tried (and tries) to be an excellent person all the time, so any failure isn't through lack of effort.'

When you step into your forties, it's like being given permission to be who you really are, says Yumi.

'A lot of us decide that we won't carry around that shame any more about being a woman — around periods, wrinkles, the fact that we have a vagina — any of that stuff.

'The way I look at it, you've got a finite amount of fucks to give. You allocate them to family and friends, but with everyone and everything else, you ration them out. You're more careful. Don't give a fuck about people you don't like, for example, and don't let people try to make *you* give a fuck about something that you don't. Give a fuck about the *right* stuff.'

The death of her father when she was 19 was a defining experience for Yumi.

'He was only 58 years old. He thought he had time, but he didn't. He was really talented as an artist but never properly pursued it. I think it was less risky to keep postponing his dreams. The things that thrilled him and gave him joy, he let go. He thought, "I'll do it later, when I've got time." It was terribly sad to witness his time run out, and I've never stopped reflecting on it.'

Seeing her father's talent remain unfulfilled was one of the drivers prompting Yumi to follow her dreams. 'When I took my first cookbook to publishers, for example, I felt invincible because I really didn't care about it being rejected. I knew I had the power to pursue this idea until it got published. I was inexhaustible.'

Similarly, it was Yumi who proposed to her husband, rather than waiting for him to take the lead.

'Even in this day and age people can't believe it. But I hit upon something when I was younger — I started asking men out and was really quite bold. We were all told that you wait for the guy to ask you out. It's so passive, so powerless. Being the active one, the asker, was a revelation — I felt like I'd unlocked the matrix for dating. If they said no, at least I'd given it a go and knew I'd hopefully given them a sincere compliment. If they said yes, I got laid.

'Make grand gestures — you really don't have anything to lose.'

▲

Celebrate You!

219

It was a win–win situation. Make grand gestures — you really don't have anything to lose.'

As the mother of four children, Yumi says the thing that makes her soul 'roar with happiness' is a bit of solitude. 'I go on vacations by myself. And yes, I could be using that money to pay off our mortgage, but I know I could be dead before I get the chance to do the thing that makes me glow, so I try to live with a bit of soulful selfishness.'

Although Yumi has worked fairly solidly since her first television presenting position in her early twenties, she understands the media's thirst for bright young things.

'It's fairly human that in the general currency of what is "cool" and cutting-edge, you're seen as less "hot" as you grow older. But there is a flipside: as you get older, you have a much clearer view of where the boundaries of knowledge and bullshit lie.

'Of course you make mistakes,' Yumi admits. 'It affects you most when you deeply hurt someone's feelings and that wasn't your intention. It can be a blow to your confidence. But stay staunch to yourself. You have to be able to filter criticism to hear what is fair and useful, and ignore what is motivated by jealousy — or something more sinister like sexism, racism or just plain boringness.

'Experience is so important,' she adds. 'It's amazing to feel like you've finally really landed in your power, and I know so many cool, inspiring and kind older women. The tide is turning, and women are really starting to back each other and form little silos of influence. If you're sick of explaining yourself, look around — you'll find your community. Luckily, women really do hit it off with each other easily. There's a real essence of humanity there, and it's the most powerful thing.'

'It's amazing to feel like you've finally really landed in your power.'

▲

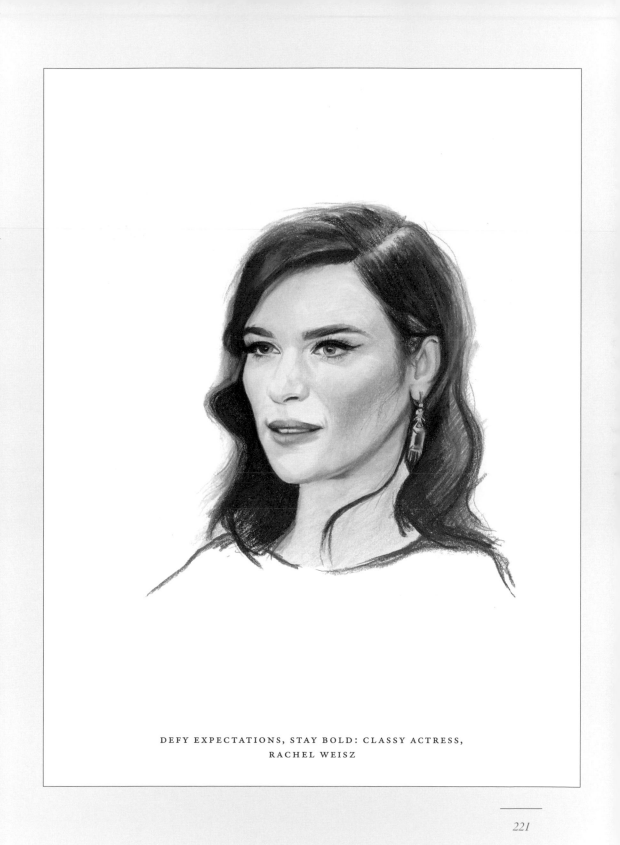

DEFY EXPECTATIONS, STAY BOLD: CLASSY ACTRESS,
RACHEL WEISZ

It's okay to disappoint people

INTERVIEW WITH BELINDA ALEXANDRA, WRITER

▲

The author of ten bestselling novels (including *The Invitation*, set in New York's gilded age at the turn of the 20th century), Belinda Alexandra says that the biggest thing life has taught her is to not take responsibility for other people's happiness — and to not make others responsible for hers. Here, she shares the joy of finding your sense of self, and stepping into your own power.

It's up to me to make myself happy, and it is up to others to make themselves happy.

A huge mistake I have made with men is to allow them to place all the responsibility on me for their happiness. The truth is, our happiness comes from our own view of the world — the thoughts and beliefs we cultivate, and the actions we take for ourselves to create the kinds of lives we want. Nobody can think anybody else's thoughts, so nobody has the power to make anybody else happy.

If I have allowed someone to make me responsible for their happiness, then guess who they blame when they are not happy?! And guess who runs around like a hamster on a wheel trying to achieve the impossible to fix the problem? Making yourself responsible for someone else's happiness means you will filter everything you do through their eyes, and that is the fastest way to lose yourself.

Taking responsibility for your own happiness is the most empowering thing you can do. In a way, you make yourself your own best friend and you get proactive about your own life.

By refusing to take responsibility for other people's happiness, you also set up really strong and healthy boundaries about what you will and will not do. As a result, you start to attract other people who take responsibility for their own happiness — and then you really start to create rewarding, reciprocal and supportive relationships.

On the other side, it's really important for women to realise that just as we are not responsible for someone else's happiness, we are not responsible for their unhappiness either. It's okay to disappoint people sometimes. We have to trust they will take responsibility for themselves and their feelings and will just get over it. If they don't, that really isn't our problem.

We need to stop feeling so guilty all the time. If you are polite and honest that is *enough*. I think women in particular are socialised to do everything we can to make others happy and to avoid making others unhappy at *all* costs. For many of us, we are socialised to be 'good', and being good is equated with being 'unselfish' — being lovely and cheerful no matter what: the gracious hostess, the woman who never swears, the woman who looks after everyone; in other words, the woman who is perfect.

One of the things I have had to switch in my mind is seeing being a people pleaser as 'good' (keeping the peace, not upsetting anybody, making sure everyone is happy, gets what they want, etc), to seeing being assertive as 'good' instead.

When you are assertive, you say what you want and think in a direct way. This allows others to speak up and say what they want, too. Then you can negotiate things that will make you both happy. Sometimes you will put someone else first, but that will be an active decision you make, and not a default position.

By being assertive and speaking up, you will let people know who you authentically are. And nothing is better than that.

'We need to stop feeling so guilty all the time. If you are polite and honest that is enough.'

▲

Celebrate You!

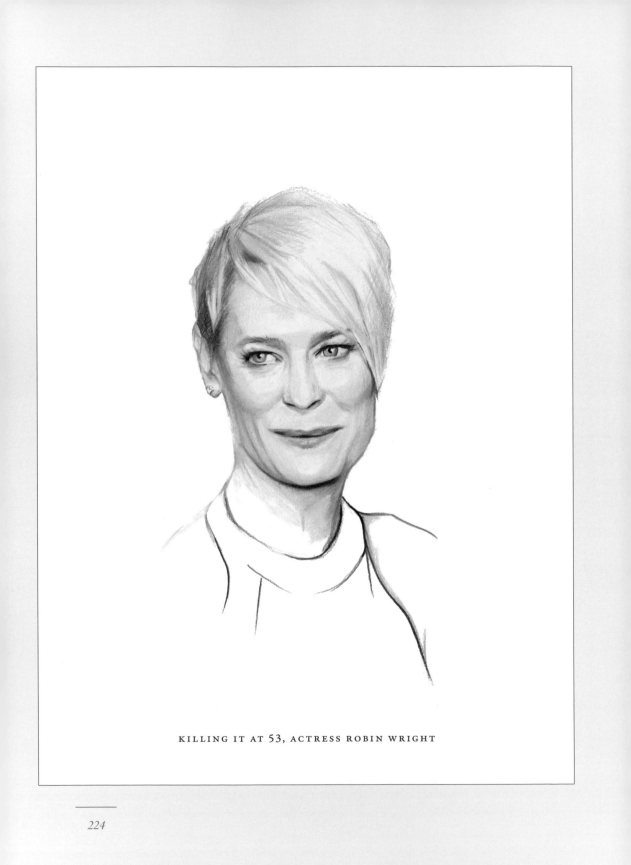

KILLING IT AT 53, ACTRESS ROBIN WRIGHT

I have finally figured out who I am

Q&A WITH CHARLOTTE SMITH,
AUTHOR AND CURATOR

▲

Charlotte Smith, 58, is the author of the bestselling books, *Dreaming of Dior* and *Dreaming of Chanel*, which include stories about many fabulous outfits and the high times spent in them — from first dates in a cheeky little 1970s minidress to mixing with the upper echelons of 1930s New York high society in a black cape for the Opera. As the curator of The Darnell Collection, a collection of over 3000 fashion items from the last century and a half, she has intimate knowledge of where these items have been worn, and by whom, and has herself lived a life less ordinary which involves travel, glamour and fashion.

What is it about growing older that brings you joy, and how do you embrace the stage you're at in life?

At 58, I have finally figured out who I am, what I believe in and what makes me tick. At last, I am at ease with being me, a phrase that is a bit clichéd, but, personally, finally reaching this point of self-acceptance has been such a great relief.

'Age' allows me to look back and reminisce about my family, adventures, friendships, opportunities, experiences, conflicts,

Celebrate
You!

beliefs, and so on. It definitely motivated me to want to discover, reflect, resolve, and change how I engage with my life in order to find a more peaceful 'me'. I wanted to become better. It was very much a personal goal. I am driven and always want to be or give 100 percent.

With the help of my sister, a health and wellbeing coach, I followed a step-by-step process of reflection and positivity. The past year and a half has been confronting, but also enlightening. I never realised how past experiences, which seemed so trivial at the time, can be catalysts for the way I react in the present. For the first time, I have learned how to step back and reassess before I react.

'Age' has motivated me to get on with it: to choose between continuing as I was, or finding a way to understand myself better so I could become the 'me' I wanted to be. I definitely feel more relaxed now as a person and, in a strange way, proud, that I have been able to figure out who I am and embrace this. It brings me a huge amount of joy.

You always seem to be travelling or doing something interesting, and I admire the wonderful energy you put into everything you do. How do you stay so vibrant and young at heart?
I get my energy from focusing on beauty. I see beauty everywhere and always try to surround myself with it. A small detail gives me as much pleasure as something huge. For me, beauty comes from being aware and observant.

My private fashion collection allows me to work with some of the most beautiful clothes ever made. The collection has taken me all over the world and has given me a chance to glimpse beauty in the most unusual places. At home, I am surrounded with antiques and paintings, which I like to think of as a souvenir of my life so far. My garden is abundant with flowers that I pick and place in vases around the house. Presentation is important. I am definitely a visual person and love pattern, texture and colour.

The
Power Age

Being inquisitive is another way I stay young at heart and is a habit I picked up from my English mother and grandmother.

I grew up surrounded by strong women and people much, much older than me. I loved their stories, their habits and their views on life. My brother, sister and I were constantly immersed in history and storytelling. We were intrigued.

My mother was a voracious reader, which ensured the bookshelves were filled with classics and books by multicultural authors. Thinking back, I remember she always seemed to have a dictionary on hand. My grandmother passed away just before her 109th birthday. Her mind was active up until the last minute. Her inquisitiveness was infectious. I loved the fact she received a BA Hons in French at Exeter University at 92, and brushed up on her Arabic at 100.

I hope I live to a nice, grand age. This means I have years of discovery ahead of me, with so much more I want to learn.

'My grandmother passed away just before her 109th birthday. Her mind was active up until the last minute. Her inquisitiveness was infectious.'

▲

How do you think we can boost our assets as we get older, both in career and relationships (either romantic or friendships)?
I have high standards for myself. I feel this reflects how I work and whom I meet. I like to be organised with a routine and use this as a structure to enable me to execute everything I do. It probably makes me sound like a control freak — which I hope I am not — but by having an imaginary bar that I can raise, I keep focused.

Just because I am older doesn't mean my standards need to drop. If anything, I love the idea I am reaching a stage when a lifetime of experiences and challenges have created the 'me' I am today, and can take me forward as a more realistic and confident woman.

I guess what I'm saying is that standards empower me, and if I am empowered I feel confident, and this is reflected in the way I interact on a daily basis. Being empowered, in turn, makes me feel good.

Celebrate
You!

How do you refuse to 'act your age'?

Age doesn't change my desire for life experiences. It just changes the type of experiences I am after.

I still lust after fabulous shoes by, for instance, Roger Vivier, but choose a shoe that suits my personal look, as a woman in her fifties rather than in my twenties. I still want to immerse myself in the beauty of another city or country — say Florence in Italy — but as a traveller who prefers a luxury stay, rather than as a wide-eyed university student content to sleep on the floor in a friend's apartment.

I still want to do everything I possibly can, but in the capacity of me being at a different stage and age in my life. This is what is so fabulous and so exciting about my future.

There are moments I honestly forget I am in my fifties and not the age of the younger people I am surrounded by. But this gets back to being passionate and having lots of energy. These two traits transcend age and help make everyone youthful.

I love hearing what young people have to say, hear their views, share their dreams. I also enjoy verbally sharing my knowledge and stories because I believe storytelling is the most powerful way of connecting. Perhaps this is because my generation relied on verbalising and communicating through words, and without sounding like a total fossil, younger generations such as my daughter's (she's 19), are accustomed to reading or watching stories unfold online.

I intend to keep my hair blonde forever more, but perhaps go from platinum to ash! I plan to wear fabulous red lipstick and to dress in a way that captures my love for clothing, rather a look that defines my age.

I want to go out and explore, to enjoy the sensation of experiencing something new, meet people, shop, and share my goals and visions. Age won't change or hamper my desire. I'll just do it with the years of reflection and experience I now have under my belt.

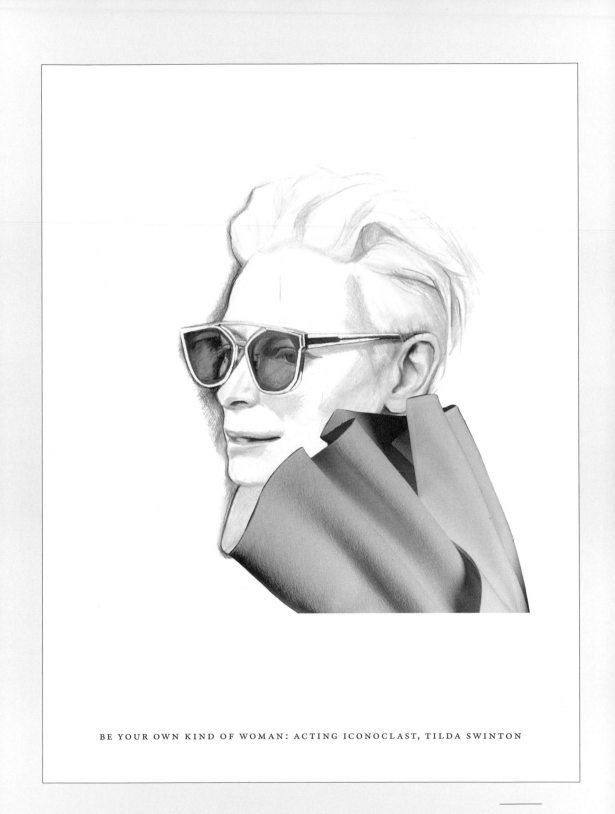

BE YOUR OWN KIND OF WOMAN: ACTING ICONOCLAST, TILDA SWINTON

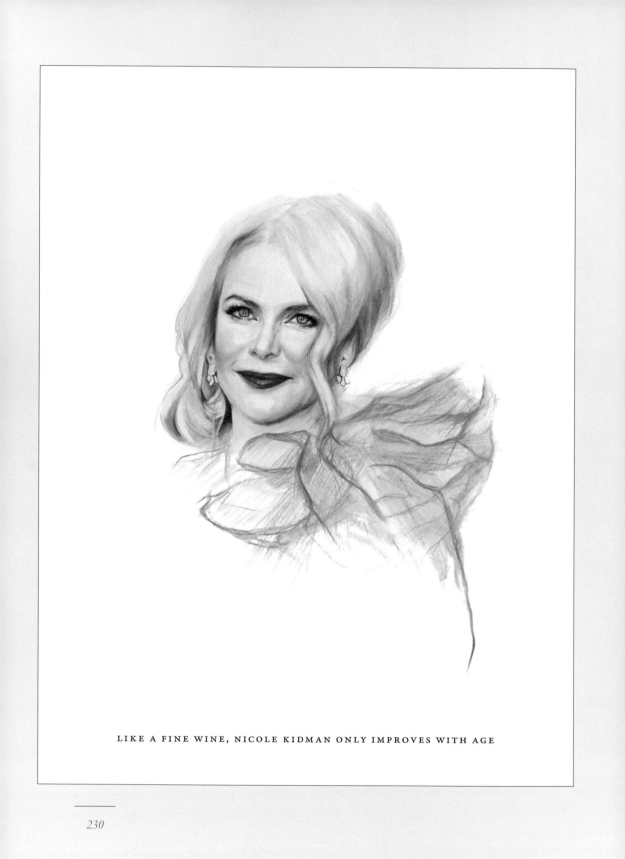

LIKE A FINE WINE, NICOLE KIDMAN ONLY IMPROVES WITH AGE

Charlotte's tips for ageing with panache

- Exude passion and a vibrancy for life. These two qualities are the great elixirs to youthfulness in older women because passion is infectious. Not only is it liberating to be passionate, but it's empowering, too, as it will attract like-minded people into your orbit.

- Dress in clothes that are vibrantly coloured and patterned, and use words that reflect the vibrancy you feel for everything you do.

- Stay in shape — exercise should be an important part of your daily routine. Pilates in particular allows you to focus on yourself while pushing your stamina to the limit.

- Well-fitting clothes make you feel confident.

- Don't deprive yourself of things you enjoy, but what I eat and drink is in moderation. Everything has to be the best quality and the healthiest I can afford. Living in France for six years made me appreciate and enjoy fine wine and champagne that enhance every meal I eat.

- Learn to accept the changes to your body and look at them as challenges rather than feeling overwhelmed. My father used to say, *For every challenge there is a solution*. In this case, the solution is called motivation.

Celebrate
You!

'ADVENTURE BEFORE DEMENTIA'

▲

This is what Kathy Lette, who recently left her partner of 28 years to take off on a gap year, says. The author of *Puberty Blues* got a shock when she realised she was about to turn sixty, and couldn't stop thinking about all the things she'd never done or seen, her mind jumping from one missed opportunity to the next.

'The great wildebeest migration in Kenya, Carnival in Rio de Janeiro, the Taj Mahal. The aurora borealis. George Clooney ... naked ... I want to swim with whales and ride a Harley. I've never been in a threesome. Hell, I haven't even played doubles at tennis!'

Announcing to her kids that she was chucking in the tea towel to globetrot for a year went down like a lead balloon — but she did it anyway. Like Shirley Valentine, the fictional bored housewife from Liverpool who takes a trip to Greece and falls in love, you can still always switch it up and change your fate.

Life is so short. Take it by the scruff of the neck and do what it is you've always wanted to do, before it's too late. Say YES to that spur of the moment vacation, to impromptu drinks with a colleague, to a spontaneous wild party. Yes can be restorative, yes can be exciting. Yes can make you feel frisky and vital again, because yes contains hope.

CONCLUSION

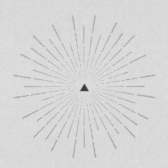

Well, here we are, and what conclusions have we reached? There is a saying that we teach what we most need to learn. Through the process of writing this book I've been seeking for myself as much as for you, dear reader, a way to move forward with grace and style and embrace this ageing lark for all its richness and pleasure and fabulousness. I hope you've picked up some invaluable insight and tips from La Que Sabe as well for luxuriating in your own power age.

Share this with your daughters, pass it on to your friends, and spread the word to anyone who will listen. Because we all need help grappling with that age-old question: how to accept our short time on this earth, when we know it will one day come to an end?

While we still breathe, there is no expiration date for living life to its fullest expression. Even in the smallest, most minuscule ways, like gazing upon the face of someone we love, revelling in glorious sunshine, or really tasting the delicious food on our plates. Or, like the 103-year-old lifetime dancer Eileen Kramer does, dancing from the waist up now that she no longer has the balance to do so standing. Where there's a will, there's a way, and doesn't that make your heart sing? It does mine.

Please don't be ashamed of your age — wear it as a badge of pride. You made it, you got there, and you're alive — not everyone is so lucky.

Life presents us with a mountain of challenges, but who would want it any other way? Don't mess about in the foothills — aim for the dizzying heights! You may not feel like you have ever reached its peak, but at least you gave it a red hot go. A big wide world — and an endless bucket list — awaits.

xo Kelly

ACKNOWLEDGEMENTS

Thank you so much to all my colleagues at Murdoch Books and Allen & Unwin who supported and made this book possible. Thank you to publishing director Lou Johnson and *The Power Age* publisher Jane Morrow for your wisdom and guidance; to editorial manager Julie Mazur Tribe and editor Katri Hilden for your expert text excising, advice and endless hard work; to Claire Grady for proofreading; to Sandy Cull, Vivien Valk and Estee Sarsfield for such stunning layout and design; to Justin Wolfers and Kaitlyn Smith for hunting out the best archival photography; to Lou Playfair in production, Carol Warwick in marketing and publicity and the entire sales team for your efforts to make this book the best it can be and spreading the word.

A massive thank you to my hugely talented friend, artist Jessica Guthrie, for her beautiful illustrations and collages, which have taken this book to a whole new level, and to Kirstie Clement for her kind endorsement and support - not for the first time.

Thank you to my husband, James, and daughter, Olive, who make life rich and worthwhile, and to the extended Doust and Jenkins clan for your love and support. Thank you to the fabulous Women of

Step into Your
Power Age

the Word: Josephine Barrett, Chris McCourt, Sarah Smith, Maggie Hamilton and Catherine Milne. You are WOW.

And to all the amazing women who shared their thoughts, experiences and advice here, I hope readers will find them as useful and illuminating as I have: Sarah Jane Adams, Jessica Adams, Maggie Beer, Chelsea Bonner, Helen Clark, Tracey Cox, Leona Edmiston, Kirstin Ferguson, Catherine Fox, Kirsten Galliott, Maggie Hamilton, Wendy Harmer, Heather Hawkins, Rebecca Huntley, Fiona Inglis, Lone Jacobsen, Jordanna Levin, Sally Loane, Dr Ginni Mansberg, Dr Joanna McMillan, Dijanna Mulhearn, Cris Parker, Gene Sherman, Charlotte Smith, Yumi Stynes, Jacinta Tynan, Kit Willow and the countless other women who chose to remain anonymous yet still appear here in spirit. My deepest gratitude.

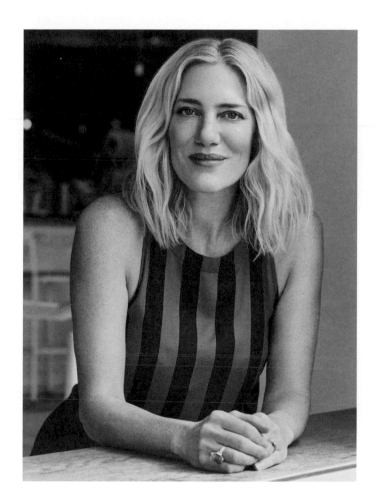

KELLY DOUST IS A BOOK PUBLISHER AND AUTHOR OF THE FASHION
MEMOIR *A LIFE IN FROCKS*, VINTAGE FASHION BIBLE *MINXY VINTAGE:
HOW TO CUSTOMISE & WEAR VINTAGE CLOTHING*, *THE CRAFTY MINX* SERIES
OF CRAFT BOOKS AND TWO NOVELS, *PRECIOUS THINGS* AND *DRESSING
THE DEARLOVES*. HER ARTICLES AND WRITING HAVE APPEARED
IN *VOGUE, AUSTRALIAN WOMEN'S WEEKLY* AND *SUNDAY LIFE MAGAZINE*.

For Murdoch Books:

Publisher: Jane Morrow
Design Manager: Vivien Valk
Editorial Manager: Julie Mazur Tribe
Designer: Sandy Cull
Editor: Katri Hilden
Production Director: Lou Playfair

Photography credits: p. 56: *Zaha Hadid Portrait* by Steve Double 01 — taken from Forgemind
ArchiMedia's photostream, flickr; p. 64: Courtesy William J. Clinton Presidential Library; p.
86: Diana Vreeland photographed in the Costume Institute at the Metropolitan Museum of Art,
1978 ©Lynn Gilbert; p. 102: World Economic Forum/Photo by Sikarin Thanachaiary; p. 127:
Yoko Ono at John Lennon Plaque Unveiling. Uploaded to 'commons.wikimedia' by Oxyman.
Author: Simon Harriyott from Uckfield, England; p. 149: From *The Algonquin Round Table
New York: A Historical Guide*, by Kevin C. Fitzpatrick, with a foreword by Anthony Melchiorri.
Published by Lyons Press, December 2014. For more information, visit algonquinroundtable.org.
Image taken from flickr; p. 152: MediaJet (A Photograph of a Photographic Portrait, captured
by MediaJet sometime in 2009); p. 164: Courtesy of Australian Human Rights Commission;
p. 172: Tina Turner in Birmingham, 2009; photo by Philip Spittle (https://creativecommons.org/
licenses/by/2.0)

Every reasonable effort has been made to trace the owners of copyright materials in this book,
but in some instances this has proven impossible. The author and publisher will be glad to receive
information leading to more complete acknowledgements in subsequent printings of the book
and in the meantime extend their apologies for any omissions.

Color reproduction by Splitting Image Colour Studio Pty Ltd, Clayton, Victoria
Printed by C & C Offset Printing Co. Ltd., China

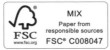